BIG GAL YOGA

POSES AND PRACTICES TO
CELEBRATE YOUR BODY AND EMPOWER YOUR LIFE

VALERIE SAGUN

D1119581

SEAL PRESS

Photography credits: All photos © Valerie Sagun except: pages 66, 188, 193, 198 © Ruel Galinato; page 12 © Jessica Rihal; page 44 © Samantha Figueroa; page 189 © Audrey Truong; front and back cover © Jennifer Anspach.

ISBN 978-1-58005-659-5
ISBN 978-1-58005-660-1 (e-book)

Library of Congress Cataloging-in-Publication Data for this book is available.

Published by SEAL PRESS
An imprint of Perseus Books
A Member of the Hachette Book Group
1700 Fourth Street
Berkeley, California 94710
sealpress.com

Note: The information in this book is true and complete to the best of our knowledge. This book is intended only as an informative guide for those wishing to know more about health issues. In no way is this book intended to replace, countermand, or conflict with the advice given to you by your own physician. The ultimate decision concerning care should be made between you and your doctor. We strongly recommend you follow his or her advice. Information in this book is general and is offered with no guarantees on the part of the authors or Seal Press. The authors and publisher disclaim all liability in connection with the use of this book. The names and identifying details of people associated with events described in this book have been changed. Any similarity to actual persons is coincidental.

Cover Design: Faceout Studios
Interior Design: Megan Jones Design

Printed in the United States of America
Distributed by Hachette Book Group

LSC-C

10 9 8 7 6 5 4 3 2 1

TO MY PARENTS, ARLENE AND REUBEN

CONTENTS

Introduction • 1

A Yogi Looks Like You! • 7

WHAT IS YOGA?

What Is Yoga? • 11

Kriya: Self-Awareness Through Ritual • 13

Jnana: Questioning to Find Self-Knowledge • 20

Bhakti: The Foundation of Self-Love • 22

Hatha: Focus on the Body • 27

Raja: The Eight Sutras • 29

Karma: Giving to Others • 31

Yoga Is for All Bodies: Beauty Standards and Big-Body Positivity • 33

STARTING YOUR BIG GAL YOGA PRACTICE

Types of Yoga • 39

Creating a Home Practice • 40

Joining a Studio • 45

Get in Gear: Yoga Clothes, Props, and Mats • 47

Get Ready to Begin: Finding Your Motivation • 58

Opening Your Practice: *Santosha* • 61

Pranayama: Yoga Breathing • 62

THE 30-DAY BIG GAL YOGA CHALLENGE

The Big Gal Yoga Challenge • 69

Day 1—Warm-Ups • 70

Day 2—Cat Pose and Cow Pose • 79

Day 3—Mountain Pose and Palm Tree Pose • 82

Day 4—Standing Backbend • 86

Day 5—Forward Fold • 89

Day 6—Low Lunge • 94

Day 7—Plank Pose and Four-Limbed Staff Pose • 98

Day 8—Cobra Pose • 102

Day 9—Child's Pose • 106

Day 10—Downward-Facing Dog • 110

Day 11—Warrior 1 and 2 • 114

Day 12—Wide-Legged Forward Fold • 118

Day 13—Chair Pose • 122

Day 14—Flow Days 1–13 Poses ▪ 125

Day 15—Extended Triangle Pose ▪ 128

Day 16—Goddess Pose ▪ 132

Day 17—Garland Pose ▪ 136

Day 18—Tree Pose ▪ 139

Day 19—King Dancer Pose ▪ 142

Day 20—Half Moon Pose ▪ 145

Day 21—Reverse Warrior ▪ 148

Day 22—Extended Side Angle Pose ▪ 151

Day 23—Bow Pose ▪ 155

Day 24—Pigeon Pose ▪ 158

Day 25—Lizard and Half Monkey ▪ 162

Day 26—Bridge Pose and Wheel Pose ▪ 167

Day 27—Half Lord of the Fishes Pose ▪ 172

Day 28—Flow Days 15–27 Poses ▪ 175

Day 29—Supine Spinal Twist ▪ 178

Day 30—Bound Angle Pose ▪ 181

You Made It! ▪ 184

More Yoga Flow Sequences ▪ 184

Aerial Yoga ▪ 187

Acro Yoga ▪ 190

YOU CAN'T CHANGE THE PAST; YOU CAN CHANGE THE FUTURE

You Can't Change the Past; You Can Change the Future ▪ 195

Don't Put Your Life on Hold ▪ 197

Conclusion ▪ 199

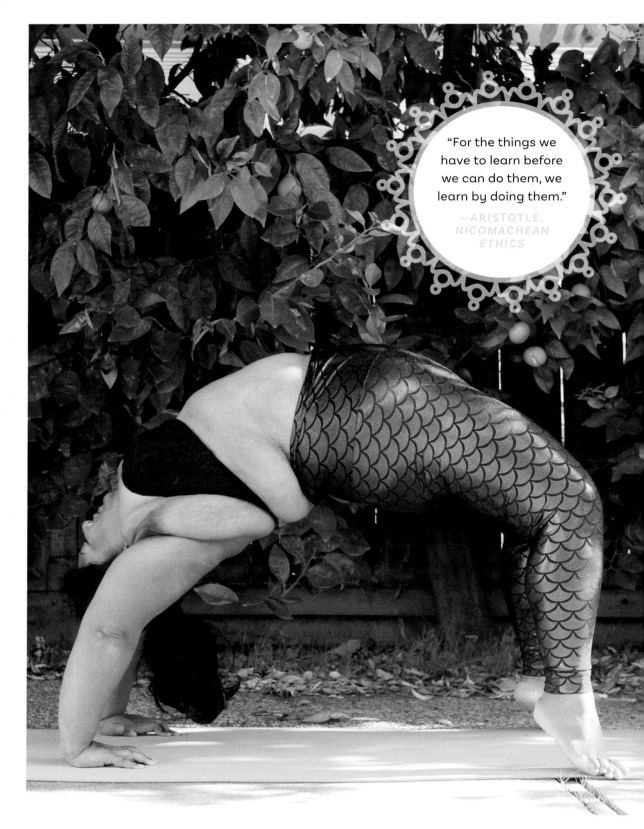

"For the things we have to learn before we can do them, we learn by doing them."

—ARISTOTLE, *NICOMACHEAN ETHICS*

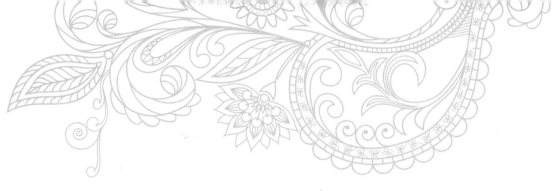

INTRODUCTION

I never set out to write a book, yet here I am! But I also never expected to be an Internet yogi with thousands of followers, or even that yoga would be a transformative part of my life. Going from being a college art student for ten years to being an Internet yogi is a drastic change of events in my life. It just goes to show that life is full of exciting and unexpected gifts we don't see coming around the corner.

So, you might be thinking, who is this big gal who does yoga? I am a big/curvy/fat woman of color, of mixed ethnicity (Asian, Pacific Islander, and Latina), who identifies with being an American, Northern Californian, middle-class, bisexual, agnostic, ambivert, and artist. My family is a mix of Filipino and Mexican, and in my hometown of San Jose—which has its own unique mix of all different ethnicities including Filipino, Mexican, Vietnamese, Indian, African American, Caucasian—I've been exposed to lots of different cultures, which has helped me to see that there isn't only one right way to do things, or one right way to be.

And while I come from and have been exposed to all of these different cultures, I don't define myself by any of them. In fact, I don't fit into any one of these slots: I'm just me. One of the reasons that yoga and its philosophy of life are appealing to me is because it fits and helps my life. My mind and body throughout my life have been open and ready for this type of practice. Yoga doesn't discriminate by attaching labels based on race, culture, sexuality, gender, or body size.

I've always been active, and most of the time my size has never limited me from trying something new. I love to swim and dance and have been doing so all my life. The truth is, our big bodies can do so much that we don't give ourselves enough credit for how powerful they can be.

When I was first introduced to yoga in college it sounded fun, especially because I've never been super-flexible. I was enrolled in the art program at San Jose State University, and at the same time I had been taking kinesiology classes, including aerobics, step, Latin dance, and swimming.

So in 2010, I took my first yoga class in college. It was a semester-long class that met twice a week for two-hour sessions. My instructor and yoga teacher was Lawrence "Lars" Caughlin. An older, slender man in his 60s, Lars was a true hippie, a nature lover, photographer, rock climber, eagle whisperer, and a dedicated yogi. When people enjoy the things they do, you can just *see* it in them—they kind of glow—and Lars glowed! I could immediately sense the way the true bliss of yoga had changed his life. He was totally magnetic, warm, and charismatic. More importantly, Lars was encouraging, and even when I struggled into a Wheel or Shoulder Stand pose, he never judged me and definitely never said anything about my weight. He always reminded me of the journey, dedication, and time that yoga requires, and the benefits that made the efforts worthwhile.

At the beginning I was definitely conscious that I was one of the two bigger-bodied people in the class. Sometimes I would look over at others and compare myself to them. Still, I'll admit that when I first started taking classes, on some level, I wanted to prove to the others that I could do whatever they could. The competitive side in me coming out! Now, I go into classes focused on my own goals, and knowing I'm content with—and proud of—all that my body can do. But back in the day, in order to be less distracted, and more motivated to learn, I started sitting up front in the class closest to Lars. That helped keep my eyes from wandering, and I could focus on my personal practice.

Over the course of the semester, as I practiced more poses and learned more about the philosophies of yoga, my interest continued to grow and I became more engaged. I found myself looking forward to the next class, practicing at home, and talking about yoga with friends. Yoga was beginning to steal my attention! Something great was happening to me, and it had to do with yoga, but I didn't quite understand it yet.

Then, one day, everything really clicked. I had walked into class feeling a little crappy. I sometimes get anxious and frustrated when things in my life are going

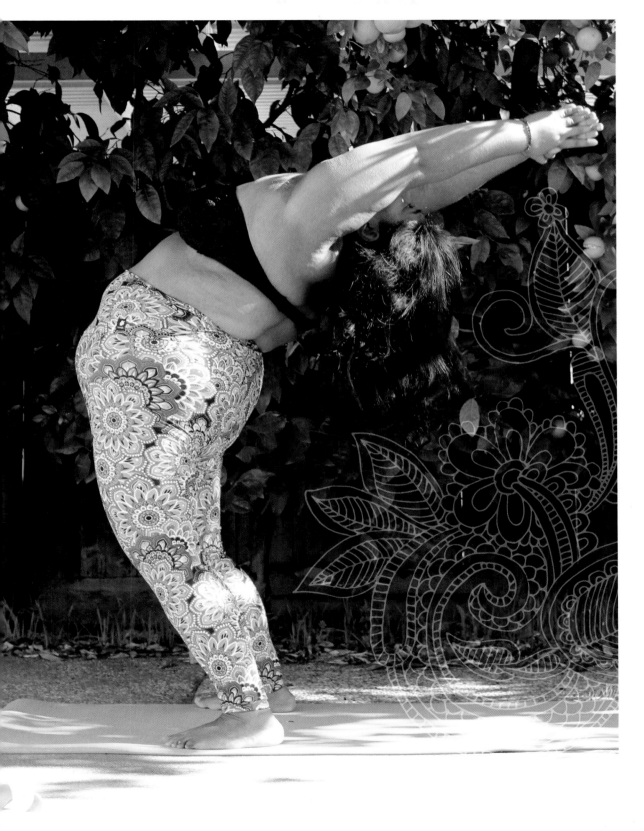

wrong, and that morning, things were definitely not going smoothly, and I was irritated. I started to go through the motions of the poses, but my heart wasn't in it. During Savasana, the final relaxation pose, I laid down on my mat, glad to be able to take a rest. As usual, I let my body sink into the floor, but this time, I somehow felt . . . different. A giant weight of negative energy lifted from me. I could actually feel my stress and frustration ease off my body. I felt not just better, but *good*. Light. Happy. When I opened my eyes I was in a completely different mood than the one I brought to class. It felt as though my mind was soaked in a soothing, calming energy. The same frustrations of my morning were still there, sure, but now the solutions were clearer, and I felt more equipped to manage my problems. I spent the rest of the day feeling elated, a sort of high I had never quite felt before. Best of all, yoga definitely made me want to try more new things, and to look at life with a more adventurous spirit!

I also began to notice that my body was changing. When I first started practicing yoga I could feel my lack of flexibility, especially in my back. But with constant practice, I definitely felt my back open, and bending became much easier. If I was struggling with a pose for a while, I realized that, with dedicated practice, eventually I would become more flexible and comfortable in that position. In general, I felt more alive than ever before.

I also began to feel stronger, especially up in my core. I'm able to do all of the poses with my bigger body because my strength and size is an asset, not a liability. You may not be able to see my strength just by looking at me, but let me tell you, it's there.

By the end of the first six months, yoga became a necessity for me; it was something that I never knew I needed in my life but now I couldn't live without it. But like everything, my motivation wasn't always front and center. Motivation is such a hard thing to find—and then keep! One of my New Year's resolutions was to do yoga every day, and I immediately did not do that at all. So I decided to create a Tumblr blog that I used as a visual diary to help motivate me to practice yoga, bike, and swim.

My original post set the tone of how I wanted my blog to work for me. I wrote about wanting to be true to myself, feel good in my own body, be physically active through yoga and swimming, and not focus on weight loss. Posting about my practice helped me to stay both on track and upbeat. As the days went by I wrote about the poses I was learning, and also about my life—my friends and family, my love of the outdoors. I posted updates about new accomplishments and exciting moments practicing new poses and learning about my body.

Tumblr provided the motivation I needed because it offered me a space to express myself, as well as check out other people pursuing their yoga practice. As I began to get comfortable with my progress, I went looking for more. The next phase in my yoga practice included yoga challenges, especially the ones I could find on Tumblr. Other yogis, like Angie of Sassy Yogi, would put up a set of poses for the month on Tumblr, and you followed along doing a pose a day. I loved the challenges, and I really loved posting my photos!

As I began to learn from others, I slowly noticed that others were following me! Before I knew it, I started posting my own yoga challenges on my Tumblr blog. From there I moved to Instagram, where I was exposed to so many more online yogis and communities. Eventually my yoga practice became more of a statement and focused beyond myself by making posts that centered around positive body image, living life as a bigger-bodied person, traveling, self- and body love, and by creating yoga challenges for myself and others, like my self-loving yogis challenge on Instagram. I started using that tag because I wanted a way for myself and others to practice self-love through yoga, rather than seeking love from someone else.

At the beginning I didn't realize that I was creating visibility for bigger bodies by posting my yoga practice. When I first started there were hardly any photos of women like me practicing yoga. So I decided to create my own body visibility. Thousands of eyes on me is still a bit daunting to think about. But my yoga photos have shown the world that big women can do yoga, and they encourage other people with bigger bodies to try yoga for the first time. When it comes to trying new physical things, we all need get over that hurdle of negative thinking and doubt we have about ourselves. Who knows? We may become confident enough to maybe even post photos of ourselves and thereby inspire others. I did it, and you can do it, too.

No matter what you look like right now, I encourage you to offer representation for everybody—and *every body*. I know that sometimes it requires bravery to stand out. But the payoff of that bravery is a melting of stereotypes and a redefinition of what a yogi looks like. And that is what this book is really all about.

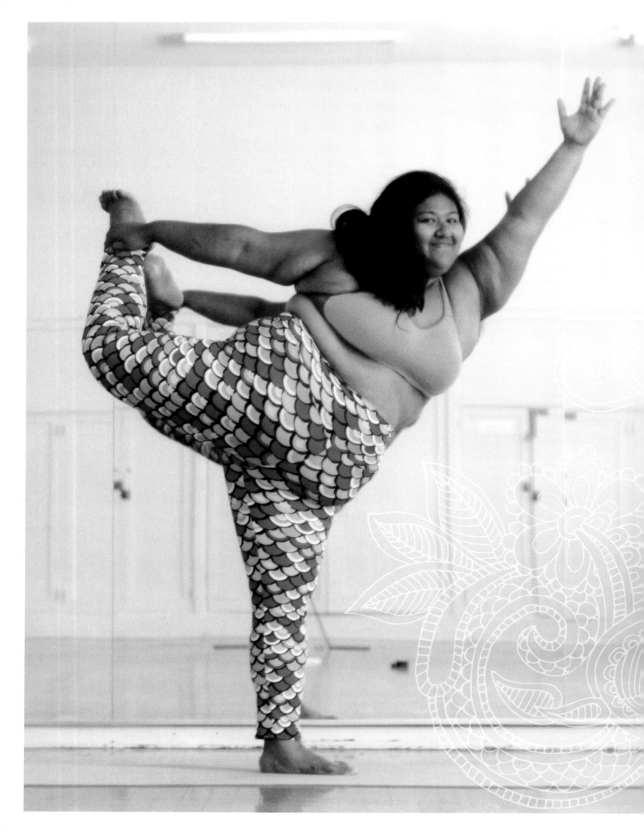

A YOGI LOOKS LIKE YOU!

'm not going to deny it; there is a real lack of representation in popular media of people that are all kinds of shapes. People of color and size often see commercials, TV shows, and magazines that pertain to white culture and are subliminally told they should aspire towards that aesthetic, even though we know that's not the real deal. In the yoga world specifically, we live in a whitewashed and weight-loss-centered universe. It's no wonder that so many believe that yoga studios are exclusively populated by thin, blonde, white women. I know that can be intimidating, because popular perception would lead you to believe you're not welcome there.

But the world in reality and online is chock full of variety. I've found others practicing yoga, both slimmer and bigger than myself, who have motivated me. My followers—many of them large women like myself—ask me all the time how to start their own yoga practice, or tell me that they were happy to see someone with my body type practicing yoga and being so open about it. I've met plenty of men and women recovering from eating disorders, thanking me for showing that there is body positivity, and finding strength in learning to love and be kind to their own bodies. I believe it's important to represent people of color in the yoga community and bigger bodies being shown as physically active without negativity. Sometimes I can't even believe that I can do that for people, and I feel very grateful and honored to be a role model that people look up to and to have created the awareness that yoga really is for everyone.

Whether you're engaging with other big yogis in a studio or online, it's all good! Together, one way or another, we'll all create a bigger yoga community. I certainly wasn't the first—Dianne Bondy, Amber Karnes, Alex van Frank, and Anna Guest-Jelley all offered specific classes for plus-size yogis. There are also plenty of yoga classes all over the country—even the world—that are designed for inclusivity. More and more studios are offering yoga classes for bigger-bodied people. Do a quick online search for "body positive yoga" or "yoga for people of color" in your area and see what's available. These classes break down stereotypes of what a yogi has to be or look like.

For me, yoga has opened the portal so that I could find my true self. It has given me the confidence to push hard even when things get rough. It has taught me to seek love for myself from myself, and not through others' approval. Yes, I still have days when anxiety or depression creeps in. But every day, despite whatever external circumstances arise, or any inner turmoil I'm experiencing, the message I tell myself—the message I have learned from yoga—is always the same: *"I am enough and I am loved."* And so are you.

Yoga accepts you as you are, and allows you to come to a space where you feel comfortable so you can connect with and learn about yourself—mind, body, and spirit. Yoga is not about an imagined version of pretty or perfect—it's about healing and honing your mind. It's about strength and flexibility, and breaking through your self-imposed mental blocks. One of the greatest gifts of yoga is that it silences the voice in your head that says, *"I can't,"* *"I am not allowed to try new things because of the way I look,"* or *"I should be ashamed/frightened/uncomfortable."* Yoga is the challenge that lets you start today, instead of telling yourself, *"I'll start when I lose some weight,"* or *"I'll never be flexible enough to even give it a try."* Remember, you do not have to already be flexible or strong to practice yoga poses. The point of the physical yoga practice is to build your flexibility and strength along your journey!

In this book, I have provided you with the essence of yoga. You will have the tools, knowledge, and awareness of the benefits yoga can bring to your life. I hope that you'll also find the acceptance you seek, and the realization that we are all perfectly imperfect. I'm excited for you to push past your self-imposed limitations and expand your mind with new challenges. So lift your body and your spirit onto your mat and feel your life take on power and purpose.

And that, my friend, takes us to where we are now. I've picked thirty of my favorite poses for you to start your own yoga practice in the form of a yoga challenge. I have found yoga challenges to be useful because when you first start out it is hard to commit to 5–30 minutes of practice per day especially with busy schedules. What is easier than committing to one pose a day to start off? As you go through the month, each day you will practice a new pose, and you can post a photo of yourself on your Instagram or Facebook accounts using the hashtag #BGYogatoEmpower in your post. This will help me to follow along on your yoga practice journey!

I know you are eagerly wanting to jump into the physical practice of yoga and start the yoga challenge right now. Don't worry, you will get there, but I believe that it is best to first understand all the different aspects of yoga beyond just the physical form. The first part of this book will help you to get the gist of what yoga is in totality and this connects to big-body positivity. In the next part, we cover different yoga types and venues, getting your gear together, motivating yourself for practice, and the basics of yoga breathing, so you will be ready to hop on your mat into your yoga challenge!

1

WHAT IS YOGA?

WHAT IS YOGA?

Well, that's a loaded question. There are so many variations of what we understand yoga to be. Is it the poses like Downward Dog and handstands? Is it meditating, breathing, chanting, eating vegetarian, philosophy, stretches? Yes, it is a mix of all of the above and much more! It is hard to pin down the full meaning of yoga as it has been brought and transferred to the Western world by gurus and teachers like Tirumalai Krishnamacharya, Swami Sivananda, B. K. S. Iyengar, Paramahansa Yogananda, and Yogi Bhajan.

The word *yoga* literally means "union" and refers to an individual's effort to become one with body and mind, with one's true self, and with truth in the world. The practice of yoga offers a way of life to encourage this union. It's a comprehensive system that incorporates breathing techniques, mantras, teachings, and—yes!—poses. So let me say that clearly: *yoga is not just about the poses.*

The *asana* (poses), which most people associate with yoga, are meant to be the gateway to the other aspects of yoga. In my experience, a lot of the other important parts of a yoga practice get pushed off to the side, and are actually the most beneficial. You can spend a lifetime understanding it all!

I think a better question is, what does yoga mean for *you?* Yoga allows me to find the time and space to perform the self-care I deserve, and as a result, to better all aspects of myself. You really have to dedicate time to practice yoga; it is a real discipline. And through the physicality of the practice I can keep my mind clear of the chaos and let go of all the ideas that clog my brain that don't aid me in life. My concerns and anxieties dissipate. When I'm off the mat, I can take my yogic outlook and see my world with a lot more clarity, so I can focus better rather than being upset with the negativity.

Yoga's philosophy involves the belief in a singular consciousness that includes each one of us. Its patterns and repetitions are meant to show us how we both belong and fit into this system of oneness in the universe. We practice yoga to remind ourselves of this deep connection and to tap into the idea that we already have within us everything we need to be happy, free, and experience joy.

To this end, there are six basic systems of yoga of which I have knowledge that are meant to open our curiosity to expose and explore our true nature. We can all

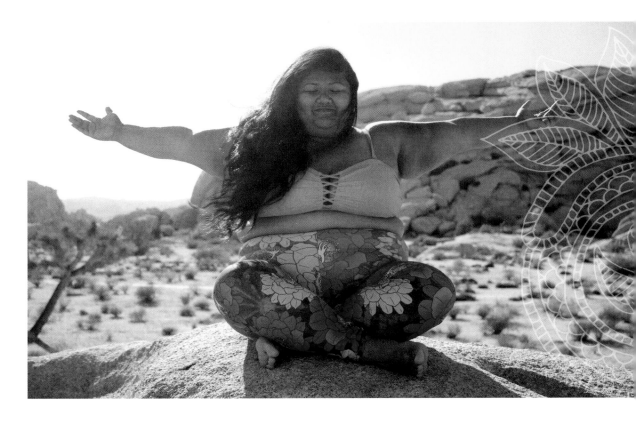

learn about these different philosophies and apply a combination of all of them to our lives. There are plenty of ways to interpret each of these core ideas, but here's how I see them:

+ KRIYA—The yoga of self-awareness through ritual

+ JNANA—The yoga of self-knowledge through deeper self-exploration

+ BHAKTI—The yoga of self-love

+ RAJA—The yoga of understanding who you truly are by way of meditation, concentration, restraint, discipline, postures, breath, attention, and bliss

+ HATHA—The yoga of the physical body

+ KARMA—The yoga of service

In the next six sections, I'll focus on each of the systems, sharing how I've incorporated it into my life and ways it can inform your practice not just on the mat, but off the mat, in your daily life. I hope that through exploring these yoga systems you can come to a place of self-love and achieve your personal goals, whether they be physical, mental, or spiritual. While you might not think that understanding these aspects of yoga will affect the way you'll do yoga on your mat, in actuality it does. Take a minute to read through and understand why yoga is so much more than any single yoga pose.

KRIYA: SELF-AWARENESS THROUGH RITUAL

Kriya Yoga includes different techniques meant to accelerate spiritual development. It is the aspect of yoga that helps us to cleanse ourselves—both physically and mentally—of negative energy using chanting, breathing, symbolic gestures called *mudras*, exercises, and physical cleanses. This is important when you have established a yoga practice because it's a way to go deeper into your practice.

The word *kriya* means "action." Each kriya is a single action that you perform repetitively to cause a predictable physiological, energetic, or spiritual outcome. Knowing what will happen when you perform a kriya allows you to have greater awareness and control over the way your mind and body function. Kriyas are the physical form of energy flow.

Kriya Yoga is therefore a practice of rituals, and there are many different types of kriya techniques. Each has a repetitious nature. For example, during my teacher training, there would be certain rituals that we would perform every day. These

"Repetition of the same thought or physical action develops into a habit which, repeated frequently enough, becomes an automatic reflex."

—NORMAN VINCENT PEALE

include chanting *mantras*, performing ritual cleanses with neti pots, and even gazing at a candle and then closing the eyes to focus on the ghost image.

Each type of kriya creates its own buzz of internal energy. Over time, as you develop more mental focus, you will become more sensitive to the subtler sensations of energy, its qualities, how it moves, and where it's blocked.

Kriya Chanting

A chant, or mantra, is a thought, word, sound, or group of words that aids in concentration and meditation. You are meant to chant the same mantra over and over, in the same tone and timing. By doing so, it creates a specific energy that you can feel on a vibrational level.

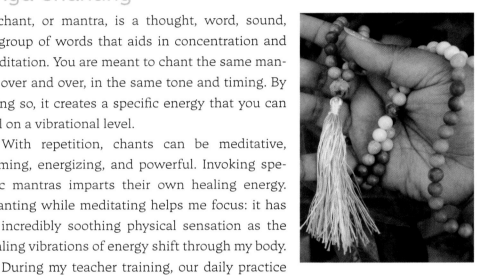

With repetition, chants can be meditative, calming, energizing, and powerful. Invoking specific mantras imparts their own healing energy. Chanting while meditating helps me focus: it has an incredibly soothing physical sensation as the healing vibrations of energy shift through my body.

During my teacher training, our daily practice started with chanting to evoke the different cosmic energies. I was new to chanting mantras, but slowly I adapted to it and found many of them to be very useful. The mantras I learned were all derived from the ancient language Sanskrit. Here are some of my favorites:

"OM KLIM SHUM SHUKRAYA NAMAHA"—VENUS PLANET MANTRA

This mantra evokes the planet Venus, which symbolizes love and the luxuries of life. I was taught this chant by my yoga teachers and told to use this mantra for myself because I tend to not let myself indulge my emotions in the areas of pleasure, beauty, and luxury, which would be beneficial for me. I still have thoughts that I do not deserve to feel joyous, even when being praised for accomplishments, which then shut down my ability to be happy and appreciative of the wonderful gifts given to me.

To change my way of thinking, and to stop berating myself, I repeated this mantra every day, at least nine times. This practice showed that I was deserving of love and beauty without judgment. I would chant it throughout the day if I felt I needed it, or chant it on Fridays, the day of the week that is intimately connected with the planet Venus.

"OM GAM GANAPATAYE NAMAHA"—GANESHA MANTRA

This mantra is for the God Ganesha, who is the remover of obstacles. It is meant to help awaken our foundation and to remove blocks that keep us from achieving a strong sense of self. I find it to be a very comforting mantra to chant in the morning because it creates a positive and uplifting energy that prepares you for the day.

"ONG NAMO, GURU DEV NAMO"

In Kundalini Yoga, a style of yoga that opens up energy channels within the body, this mantra is the opening chant that is used in place of saying Om during a regular yoga class. It translates to "I bow to the creative wisdom, I bow to the Divine Teacher within." This chant evokes the divine wisdom of the universe and self-knowledge within us. Even though this is a chant better used in a class, it is still one of my favorites. When there are times that you need to look within yourself, this is a great mantra to chant.

"RA MA DA SA, SA SAY SO HUNG"

This is another healing chant used in Kundalini Yoga. As you say it, you are sending positive energy from the chant out to people who need it. It invokes the sun, moon, earth, and universal energies for healing within the self or sending to others. The first time I tried this mantra, I actually cried while reciting it during a class with Gurmukh Kaur Khalsa. I broke down, wanting to heal everyone who has expressed or is silently struggling.

"LET GO"

A chant that I have been working on for myself is the mantra "Let Go." It is a simple mantra, but it's very powerful. I have a hard time letting challenges, negative thoughts, and difficult people go. This is a good mantra to practice when you need to take a moment to clear away frustrations that are clouding your judgment.

Kriya Cleansing with a Neti Pot

Another example of a kriya is using a neti pot (Jala Neti). This kriya is more than a ritual, because it's really a physical cleanse for your sinus cavities. At the same time, it offers a way to physically cleanse you of thoughts, ideas, and habits that you're trying to get rid of.

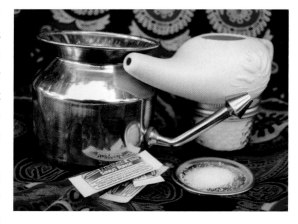

I've come to really love using a neti pot because I tend to have sinus congestion, and it flushes out excess mucus and prevents irritation. A neti pot can look like a teakettle with a long spout. It can definitely seem intimidating and strange, but I promise that it doesn't hurt, it's simple to use, and it's beneficial. I have two neti pots, a big metal one and a smaller one for when I travel. They are so commonly used now that you can pick one up at almost any drugstore or online.

The solution to fill the neti pot should be warm, not hot! You don't want to hurt yourself. Use cool filtered or purified water mixed with boiled hot water and sea salt—a full teaspoon with a bigger neti and a half teaspoon with the smaller neti. Stir the water until the salt is fully integrated. (You can also purchase packets of prepackaged solutions online and at market or drug stores.) When you're ready, here's what you'll do:

+ Find a comfortable position. When I first started I found that a squatting position was most comfortable if you are using it outside. Or, you can bend over a sink, or in the shower. Water will be streaming out of your nose, so wear appropriate clothing wherever you do it.

+ Tilt your head sideways so that your nostrils lie one over the other. This will help the flow of water to work with gravity as it moves out the lower nostril.

+ Insert the neti spout in the top nostril with the pot in an upright position so the water is not flowing out. You do not need to shove the spout all the way into your nose: it just needs to be in far enough to create a seal so the water does not leak out.

+ Start to tilt the neti so that the water streams in through the top nostril, giving it some time to pour out of the bottom nostril. Usually the first nostril takes longer because it is cleaning out most of the mucus. Breathe through the mouth calmly to prevent from snorting the water into the nasal cavity. Water may start trickling down your throat, and that's okay just spit it out and keep going. This process can take some time to be comfortable. You are learning how to make it feel natural and flow freely for you. Play around with it, adjusting the tilt of the head and tilt of the neti.

+ Repeat the procedure on the other nostril, turning your head so that the bottom nostril is now on top.

+ Once you are finished with both sides it is important to get rid of the excess water. If there is too much solution left in the nasal cavity, it can dry it out and cause problems. To get rid of excess water, bring the head back up to an upright position. Place a finger over one nostril, blowing gently but forcefully out the opposite nostril. Water and mucus will be coming out, so have a towel or tissues handy. Blow out ten times on each side, and then ten times out both nostrils at the same time.

+ When you are finished, stand up tall, feet apart from each other, raising your arms up overhead. Bend the knees, and sweep your arms forward and down in a quick motion, blowing out through both nostrils. Repeat ten times, and on the last one hang out in a Forward Fold (see page 89), letting the remaining water drain out of your nose.

✦ Repeat if you want to make sure you got all of the solution out of your nasal cavity.

Kriya Poses

Kriya poses are not just one specific posture most of the time. They are a series of exercises usually involving dynamic movement. This helps to build up positive energy that then releases negative dormant energy. The following are a few Kriya exercises that I like to practice regularly. Your breath through these specific poses should be a short forceful sniff in and out through the nose.

SITTING AS THE TORSO MOVES BACK AND FORTH—Sit in a comfortable position on the floor or chair with the spine upright. Place the hands onto the tops of the knees. Keep the head steady with the chin parallel to the floor. Inhale; round the back bringing center of the back behind you. Exhale; push the chest forward. Find your own rhythm and pace inhaling and exhaling as you move the spine back and forth. Let the hands stabilize you keeping the head upright. This is a simple exercise to help warm up the spine. Repeat for one minute.

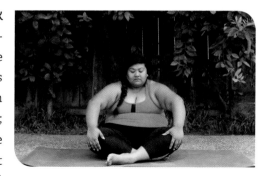

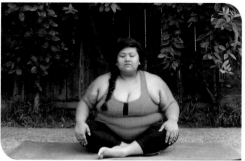

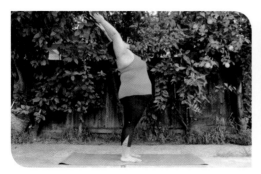
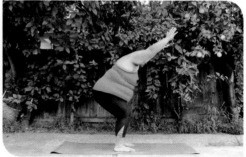
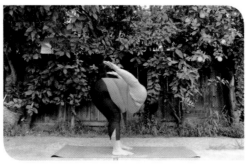

STANDING BACKBEND UP AND DOWN TO FOLD FORWARD—Begin standing with feet hip-width apart. Inhale, reaching the arms up overhead and reaching backward, bend the knees, and exhale as you sweep the arms forward and down, then back behind you as the torso folds over the thighs. Inhale; sweep the arms up lifting and engaging the lower back to come back up, and taking a slight backbend as the knees straighten. Repeat this movement going up and down at your own pace for one minute.

SEATED WIDE-LEGGED, BOWING WITH HANDS BEHIND THE HEAD—Take a seat down on the floor or chair with the legs out wide. Place the hands interlaced behind the base of the skull, forearms parallel, and elbows out. Inhale, and then exhale hinging at the hips fold forward bringing the forehead towards the floor. Inhale, lift back upright, and exhale to fold forward again. Repeat for 1 minute at your own pace.

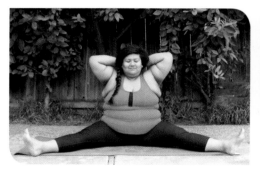 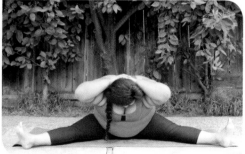

These are just a few of many different types of kriyas. A yoga practice that works with kriyas is Kundalini Yoga.

JNANA: QUESTIONING TO FIND SELF-KNOWLEDGE

Jnana is a yoga practice that takes place off the mat. Jnana is a philosophical part of yoga that puts you on the path of wisdom and self-knowledge by having you practice self-questioning, reflection, and intellectual enlightenment as you investigate your thoughts, identity, and ego. It is a formal way to develop deep inquiry and personal contemplation so that you can work out who you are and who you want to be. Ultimately, it allows you to be your highest self by understanding perception, detachment, calmness, control, truth, and concentration.

Self-knowledge doesn't occur with one "eureka" moment. Instead, it's a daily challenge of self-questioning. Every day I strive to do things to better myself, but if you try to force a whole different lifestyle in one go, chances are it will only end up being a phase for you. Take time to get to know what you are like and who you are, and enjoy the ongoing process of exploring yourself.

Within Jnana, there are four attributes, which indicate avenues of self-knowledge. One of them that is easier to approach is called Viveka, which is to distinguish intellectually between what is real and what is not real. It is finding the "right understanding" of the Self and non-Self, long term (eternal) and short term (temporary), pleasure and bliss, and the truth and soul versus materiality. According to Yogapedia, "Viveka is an important aspect in the physical practice of yoga as well. It shows one's skill in discerning the details in one's alignment, by turning one's attention inward and working with the invisible details. Learning to detect the details about one's yoga practice helps to improve the practice itself, but can also increase the quality of 'off the mat' experiences as well."

Jnana Helps You Discover What You Really Love

I've used Jnana to follow the passions that shape my personality and provide a form of self-expression. Doing what you love helps you to better know you.

What are your passions? What excites you? What intrigues you? A passion doesn't need to be grand or glorious—it could be a hobby or personal interest. Do you knit, read, sing, cook?

A passion can be the way you spend your time—with friends and family, pampering yourself, or traveling. These are all wonderful ways to love what you're doing and learn about yourself at the same time. When I'm doing what I love, I feel dedicated to the process, and I'm putting my whole heart into what I'm doing.

Your interests and passions can change over time, and that's not only normal, it's expected. In fact, that's when you learn more about who you are. For example, soon after I started practicing yoga I fell into a rut with my artwork. My work wasn't conveying my ideas, and as a result, I became increasingly frustrated. So I took a break from art and turned my full attention to yoga with the guidance of Jnana: asking myself "Who am I?" and finding my own "right understanding" for what I needed for myself. Question yourself about your own experiences and realities. There is not one way to figure out Jnana. It is something that cannot be taught or given, like all of yoga, because it all is based on an individualized thought process.

✦ Who am I?

✦ What is my relationship with my body?

✦ What am I doing to better my life?

BHAKTI: THE FOUNDATION OF SELF-LOVE

The underlying concept of Bhakti Yoga is love for yourself. If you don't have this foundation, then everything else about yoga is meaningless, because you cannot be positive and kind to yourself without self-love.

Bhakti is also known for encouraging a devotion to God. Personally, it's hard for me to believe in the bigger picture of who or what "God" is. However, I like the definition of bhakti that Sianna Sherman, a senior Anusara Yoga teacher, gives in *Yoga Journal:* "For me, bhakti means whatever strikes your heart with beauty, whatever hits the mark of your heart and inspires you to just feel the love." In this context, "God" is the devotion and love you have for yourself, as well as selfless love for others.

Following the bhakti path means caring for yourself as though you are precious—and you are! For me, self-love has been a learning and healing process. You have to understand yourself inside and out so that you can start loving yourself. One of the easiest ways to get to know yourself better is through self-care. In fact, I see self-love and self-care as two sides of the same coin.

Practicing self-care and self-love is especially important for those who live in big bodies. We're taught from childhood that we should get rid of even the slightest hint of fat. Unless we're skinny, we're supposed to hate our bodies and hate ourselves for letting ourselves be this way. That is mentally toxic and exhausting. And has always been the wrong approach to change.

I've heard my share of negative comments over the years while being highly visible online. I've been lucky, however, because there have only been a few instances in my life where people have made an issue about my weight to my face.

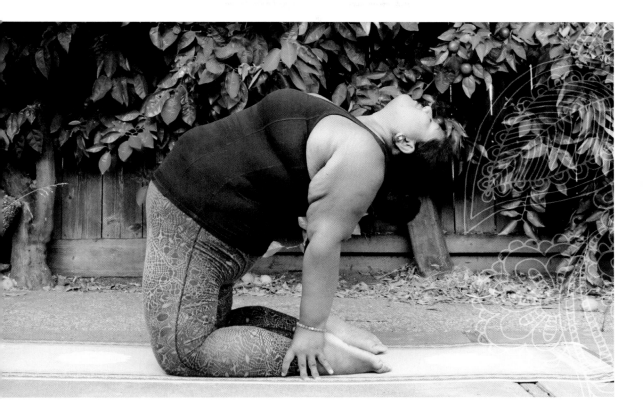

Honestly, the last time I can even remember being teased about my weight was in elementary school.

The trolls online tend to hurl generic insults like, "You're fat." Well, that's pretty much stating the obvious! Yes, I am fat, what about it? So clever *and* original, right? Sometimes they might just post a phrase like "disgusting," or more elaborate comments such as, "Why are you promoting obesity?"

All of this is generally pretty hilarious to me because I can easily dismiss it. I can honestly say, even though I can get a little obsessed with reading the comments and debating with people, on the whole I like to just laugh at how moronic people can be when they are trying to be mean. For one thing, they don't know me just because there are pictures on Instagram. Nor do they take the time to understand anything about who I am or what I promote. Therefore, I don't take them seriously and they have absolutely no power over me. I view this negative speech as toxic thinking that others don't understand they are doing.

Yoga has taught me that every body is meant to be loved and respected as it is now. You are already worthy of love. You are enough. We're all enough. Bigger bodies are just like anybody else; we just happen to have a bit more fat. We're still human. We're still people.

It's taken me a lifetime to accept all the parts of my body—lumps, rolls, scars, dark spots, uneven skin, stretch marks, fat, body hair, dry/oily skin. My body once made me upset, but now I know it's what makes me who I am in the most concrete sense. I love my body for being the home to my soul.

It feels good to have an open relationship with your body, respecting it enough to not go looking for every flaw to try to some-how "fix" it. More often than not, as long as our bodies are moving, living, passionate, and functioning, it's our minds that are getting in the way of our self-appreciation.

> "You, yourself,
> as much as anybody
> in the entire universe,
> deserve your love
> and affection."
>
> —BUDDHA

I'm not saying that I'm 100 percent happy with my body all the time. But I try not to be too hard on myself. I take au-thor Lesley Kinzel's advice to heart when she writes, "Sometimes, loving your body is not an op-tion. Sometimes, the best we can do is accept our bodies as the changeable, beau-tiful, frustrating vessels they are. That's OK. Expecting yourself to have a full-on love affair with your body at all times is asking too much. Bodies are occasionally annoying. What we can do is know them, and decide for ourselves when they feel good, and when they feel less good, and what we might do to make them feel bet-ter again. Even if we can't love our bodies, we can make sure we don't hate them."

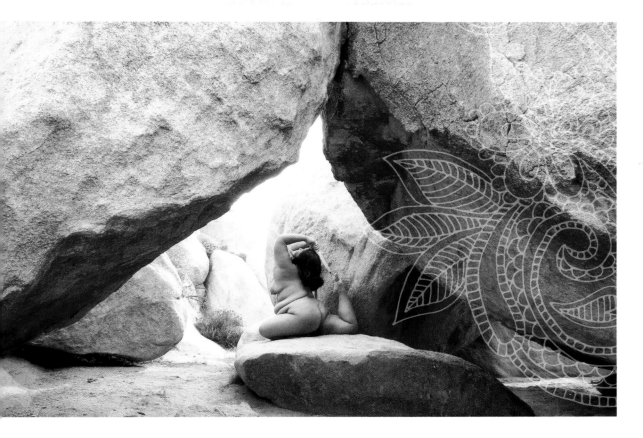

Chub Love

Here's a challenge: try yoga in just your underwear. I mean it! There is something about doing yoga in your undies or even in the nude that feels exciting. This is especially true for us big yoga gals. I thank the amazing Jessamyn Stanley, badass fat femme and fellow curvy yoga teacher, for exposing me to the idea that a big woman could practice in her undies! I had no idea how liberating it would be until I tried it for myself. On a last-minute trip to Joshua Tree National Park I went for it, and I went all the way. Keeping an eye out for wandering hikers, I took off all my clothes and went into a One-Legged King Pigeon Pose butt naked. It was extremely liberating! You don't have to streak in public, and you don't have to do anything you don't want to do. But if you want to do yoga wearing your undies, or less, just find a place in which you feel safe and comfortable. I do recommend taking a photo or two, or at least having a mirror nearby. You can start by wearing whatever you want and remove clothing as you become more confident. Look at your body in the mirror, search out every curve, and appreciate it by giving it some love. This exercise is a good way to recognize and embrace the beautiful imperfections that make your body yours.

Bhakti and Intimacy

Ultimately, bhakti and self-love are really about building body confidence and allowing yourself to be vulnerable. I used to be weirded out at the thought of other people seeing my body, because for the longest time I had been the only one to see it. My first sexual relationship was when I was twenty-six, and I remember feeling discouraged up until that point. It wasn't really that I was ashamed of my body; the discomfort derived more from the idea of letting someone else see me in an intimate and vulnerable way. When I had finally had the experience of having someone seeing my naked body, it gave me confidence to just be myself from then on. I thought to myself, *"Okay, that experience wasn't as bad as I thought it was going to be."*

Today, being naked in front of another person feels like a positive affirmation from my body to the world. I am a woman who is not afraid to embrace all that I am. My body, and bodies like mine, will be seen and not hidden from the world. We are built to connect with one another, and we should enjoy seeing each other and letting ourselves be seen!

It's wonderful to share love with others, but remember that the person we all should love the most is ourselves. This can be asking a lot of us—loving yourself is a never-ending journey. Keep working at loving yourself while loving someone else and the love will grow.

#selflovingyogis

Sometimes we can't be strong and confident in ourselves no matter how hard we try. When I needed a way to push myself in a positive way, I made the "selflovingyogis" hashtag and Instagram yoga challenge as a way of coping with memories of an ex that I was having a hard time shaking. We'd met in February the year before, and as January came to a close, I couldn't help but be reminded of him. Plus, Valentine's

Day pretty much dominates the first half of the month with constant reminders of the joys of having a significant other. I didn't want to spend my time in a funk, so I made that hashtag and hosted a last-minute, 14-day yoga challenge on Instagram. The challenge was to increase self-love for myself and others, either on the mat or off, by asking participants to honor themselves and those they love, even if those loved ones weren't romantic partners. In the challenge I asked fellow yogi participants to complete a pose a day for each of those fourteen days and post it with a caption about something that they loved about themselves, whether it was a part of their body or something that they do, or some weird little quirk. It was a way to encourage myself and others to find the love physically through a yoga practice and within themselves rather than seeking it elsewhere.

HATHA: FOCUS ON THE BODY

Hatha Yoga is the physical embodiment of yoga. It focuses on the postures—or *asana*—as well as breathing to prepare the body for meditation and achieve bliss. With the popularization of yoga through the west, Hatha has come to mean the focus on the physical poses.

The word *hatha* is a combination of *ha* (sun) and *tha* (moon), the two opposite energies that regulate the body. Working with the physical body through breathing exercises and the postures raises your yogic energy. The postures help you strengthen and tone your muscles. But more importantly the balance of Hatha helps to open the chakras, or energy centers, within the body. There are seven main chakras, and when those are stimulated, they help to create a positive energy flow. Moving the body keeps the energy from becoming static. While it is true that Hatha Yoga is the physical side of yoga, it is not

"Yoga is a light, which once lit, will never dim. The better your practice, the brighter the flame."

—B. K. S. IYENGAR

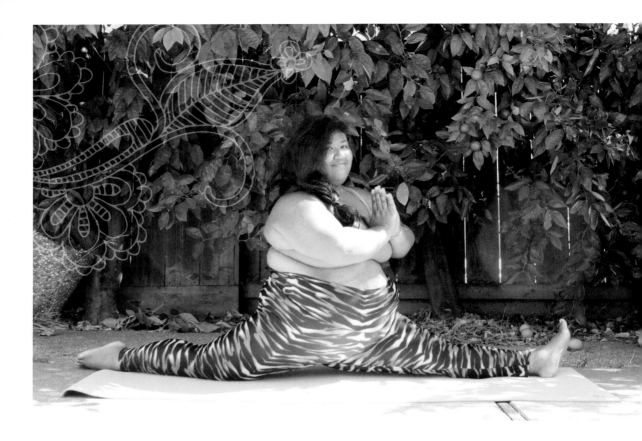

about weight loss. In my yoga practice I never was looking to use it for weight loss. I just wanted to feel good in my body as I am now. With yoga, my body is better able to maneuver, and it feels more flexible and agile. I've also become more in tune with all parts of my body, whether it's my fingers, internal organs, or legs. This has made me more aware of my body so I can take better care of it.

Hatha Yoga and Mental Health

My Hatha Yoga practice has become a type of mental health therapy for me. I have always wanted to find balance in my life, and Hatha is that balance of the sun and moon, feminine and masculine, conscious and subconscious, hot and cold, past and future. By focusing more on the present and balance during my practice, I can let go of the mental blocks that haven't been helping, or have actually been holding me back. That doesn't mean that there is a magical quality to yoga: my struggles are still there; I just have a better way of assessing them, and ultimately, of dealing with them, often by finding the happy medium in between. I can say that overall, I've been able to let go of the anger and negativity that I was attaching to my personal problems.

For instance, part of my journey has been dealing with depression. Depression itself is a beast; managing it is a daily battle. I've sunk to low points where I felt like I was stuck in a hole trying to dig my way out, but kept sliding back no matter how hard I tried. It felt like there was no solution. On some of the worst days, I just wanted nothing more than to hide under the covers, cry, and eat.

In the past, the best I could do was to keep hoping that things would get better. But once I started becoming more aware of how I felt in the present, and stopped dwelling on the past and giving myself anxiety about the future, I realized that even a tiny bit of self-care goes a long way. When I got caught in a cycle of anxiety and depression, I would do yoga, and then I'd do self-care that I would enjoy, like put on some cute lingerie, a cute dress, or binge watch *The Walking Dead*. I still couldn't get over my negative feelings completely, but slowly my decision to be kind to myself chipped away at the negativity and sadness after physically activating my body.

RAJA: THE EIGHT SUTRAS

Raja (or Royal) Yoga is the complete path of introspection. We all have goals that we want to achieve and ways we want to improve ourselves, whether that's gaining confidence or finding inner peace. Raja Yoga is a structure in which we can set our best intentions, achieve our highest consciousness, and try to build a meaningful life around the yogic philosophy.

Raja Yoga involves eight limbs, or *sutras*, transcribed by ancient scholar Patanjali, which are the different limbs on the yogic path to reach the final limb. As you practice each you are focusing your attention on the root of your being, becoming the person you are truly meant to be. When I first started my yoga practice I was aware of this path, but it took time for me to fully understand the meaning behind all of the sutras.

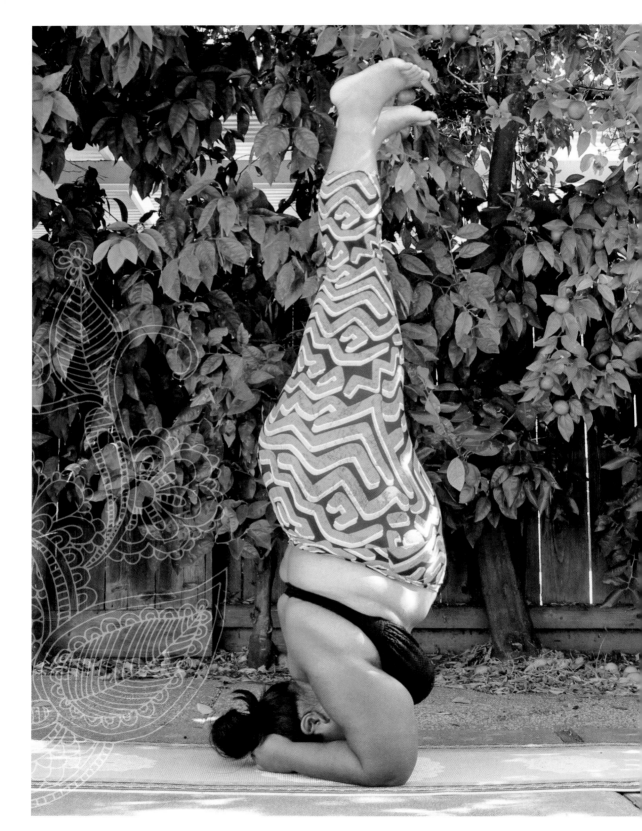

The eight limbs are:

+ *Yamas*—Morality

+ *Niyamas*—Disciplines

+ *Asana*—Postures

+ *Pranayama*—Control of breath

+ *Pratyahara*—Withdrawal of the senses

+ *Dharana*—Concentration

+ *Dhyana*—Concentration meditation

+ *Samadhi*—Bliss

Raja Yoga strings these concepts together, creating a set of guidelines for how to live. However, while the eight-limb path is guiding us, its lessons are simply something we are striving for. We are not expected to master all of them, just keep them constantly in mind so that we can apply them to different parts of our lives.

We typically skim the surface of our problems, without trying to fully understand the inner workings of our own selves. The eight limbs offer another way to look within yourself and be able to understand yourself more. By doing so, you'll have a higher level of consciousness.

You know you're practicing Raja Yoga when you start to apply these ideas to little parts of your life. Being truthful, having a sense of control, finding contentment, knowing yourself, and having compassion for others are all hallmarks of Raja Yoga.

KARMA: GIVING TO OTHERS

Karma is the yoga of service to humanity. It is the act of performing good deeds selflessly. It's a way for you to give what you can, just for the pure pleasure of giving. To that end, there is no physical reward of karma. You're not supposed to expect anything from it.

For me, I enact my karma by giving what I can to others through my yoga teaching and body positive activism. I realized a long time ago that my posts weren't just

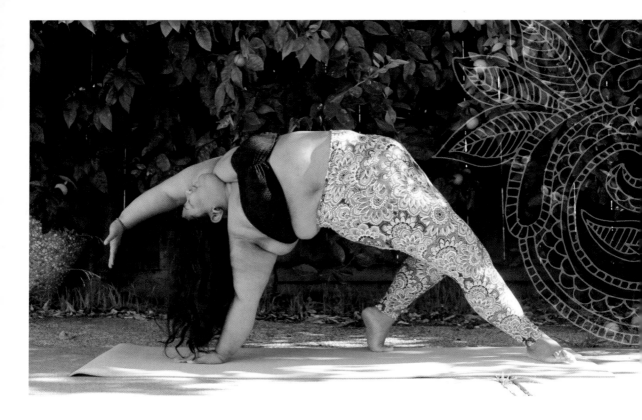

for me, or about me. It's about us, creating a community of big bodies and women of color. I was unknowingly helping other women discover the beauty of their bodies just by making myself visible through social media. Whether or not my actions affect my future, they affect others positively, and I just want to give what I can. I'm not seeking the validation of someone sending me a post saying, "Oh my God you're so great, you're an inspiration." That's very flattering and nice, but really, I'm happy just being here for you.

Altruistic acts are fulfilling. They make us better people. That's because karma is meant to help subdue the idea of the ego. The ego's singular focus can be both good and bad. It defines each of the parts of us: it is the "I" in, *"I am brown, fat, and queer."* But if we only use our ego as validation, it sets us apart from others, and in yogic terms, takes us away from the oneness of the universe. When we focus instead on the "we" instead of "me" we are letting the ego go and are able to work for more than just ourselves.

The ego is rampant on social media, where people post stuff purposely looking for fame and popularity, as if to say, *"Ooh, look at me, look at what I'm doing."* We all need to take a step back and see how this is affecting the way we think about ourselves, and others.

Selflessness Is Sharing

You can begin to selflessly give back to others when you change your view and embrace karma. Not all gestures have to be grand. They can be as simple as being kind to one another, or doing volunteer work in your community. Teachers in all kinds of fields are my inspiration for karma. We all have something to teach; find out what you want to share, and then find your audience.

YOGA IS FOR ALL BODIES: BEAUTY STANDARDS AND BIG-BODY POSITIVITY

I am a beautiful, smart, strong, and talented woman who happens to be fat. I do not subscribe to the notion that there is only one standard of beauty and one standard yoga body, and these certainly don't revolve around being thin. When I practice yoga at a studio, I look around the room and see bodies that are all different shapes and sizes, and they're all beautiful. I decided long ago that I'm not going to compare myself to anybody else because I'm good, just the way I am. Yet too many women and men believe that we have one body standard in America. They are constantly comparing themselves to others, thinking, *"I have to look like this celebrity"* or *"I won't be happy until I lose weight and look like that."*

It's time to stop this ridiculous thinking. In reality, we have millions of different bodies in all sizes and shapes. And we're all unique, just the way we are. We don't have to keep aspiring to be something that we aren't or never will be. The body that you bring to the mat is your yoga body. We don't need to conform to a certain look or aesthetic to practice yoga. Some bodies aren't labelled as "beautiful" in the media. Beauty is not associated with thinness, just like ugliness is not associated with fat. What's more, beauty standards change—all the time. All of a sudden someone comes onto the scene and changes the trend. Then, everyone wants *that* certain type of beauty. Celebrities like Jennifer Lopez were made fun of for having a naturally big butt and people still thought big lips, big boobs, and big asses were embarrassing. Yet now some women aspire to have those features, even going so far as having surgical procedures to be more curvaceous! Once some white celebrity popularizes it, then everyone suddenly changes their opinion. Then it's all about the big boobs, tiny waist, and a big ass.

"It is better to live your own destiny imperfectly than to live an imitation of somebody else's life with perfection."

—BHAGAVAD GITA

Many popular white American media co-opt then claim as their own the looks of many different cultures, including hairstyles, outfits, and accessories that are traditionally popular with black, Latin, and Asian cultures, without giving respect back to the original culture.

So let's just get this totally straight: body diversity is amazing! Why would we even want to live in a boring, cookie-cutter world, where everyone is exactly the same?

Mainstream media promote an unrealistic beauty standard by featuring thin white women almost all the time. But we are a melting pot, and the Internet provides so many more images than what we can find in magazines or on television. We can create our own visibility through our individual social media feeds, and show the world all types of beautiful women in all sizes, colors, and features.

Looking for beautiful big bodies and a diverse community of bodies? Try these wonderful pages:

+ Be the Change Yoga and Wellness
+ Wear Your Voice
+ The Adipositivity Project

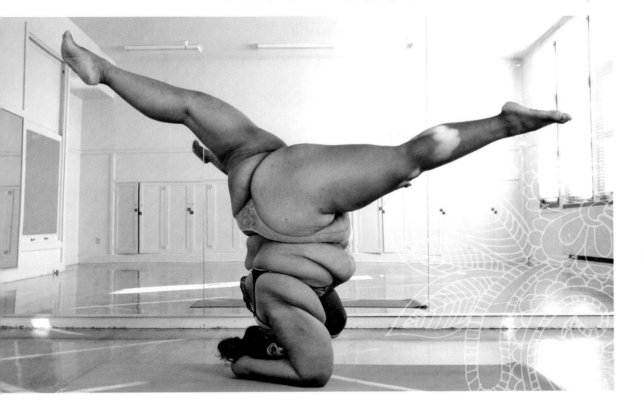

- ✦ The Body Positive
- ✦ Curvy Girl Lingerie
- ✦ Yoga and Body Image Coalition
- ✦ Yoga International
- ✦ Eff Your Beauty Standards
- ✦ The Body Is Not an Apology
- ✦ Yoga of Color

You can also follow the Instagram postings of strong women who revel in their body positivity:

- ✦ Amber Karnes—@bodypositiveyoga
- ✦ Anna Guest-Jelley—@curvyyoga
- ✦ Annie Carlin—@supportiveyoga
- ✦ Alex van Frank—@alexyvf

- Aarti Olivia Dubey—@curvesbecomeher
- Dana Falsetti—@nolatrees
- Dianne Bondy—@diannebondyyoga
- Jessamyn Stanley—@mynameisjessamyn
- Jessica Rihal—@round_the_way_gal
- Naomi Finkelstein—@practice_radical_self_love
- Rachel Estapa—@rachelestapa
- Jes Baker—@themilitantbaker
- Virgie Tovar—@virgietovar
- Chrystal Bougon—@curvygirllingerie
- Rachel Otis—@somewhere_under_the_rainbow
- Tess Holiday—@tessholiday
- Gabi Gregg—@gabifresh
- Ashley Nell Tipton—@ashley_nell_tipton
- Gloria Shuri Henry—@glowpinkstah
- Jazzmyne—@jazzmynejay
- Megan Jayne Crabbe—@bodyposipanda
- Laura Burns—@radicalbodylove

When you enter a yoga studio, try to leave your comparison mind-set behind. Don't worry if you don't look like somebody, or everybody else. There's nothing wrong or weird about you, and if there are people who will judge you, that's their karmic problem.

If you can walk into a studio and not give a shit about doing anything other than yoga in the class, you'll naturally stop worrying about being the fattest person in the room.

That's not to say that it can be very discouraging for a big gal to walk into a studio and feel underrepresented. But at the same time, you're paving the way for the next big gal. I definitely was one of few bigger bodies attending yoga when I first started and still am most of the time, but it didn't discourage me from trying yoga; it only made me want to prove myself more.

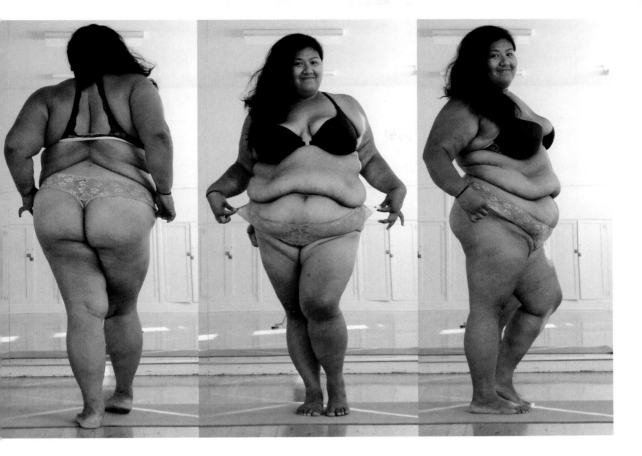

I hope that in the future, yoga teachers and classes will become more and more inclusive of different types of bodies. Teaching yoga should be about more than guiding students through a routine; teachers should also offer guidance and individual attention, not only related to size. Some bodies need adjustments for balance or injuries.

Let's break the stereotype. You are more than capable of being big and wanting to be active, without having to worry about how you look in class, or focusing on weight loss. Yoga is beneficial to you in this moment, and in your current body.

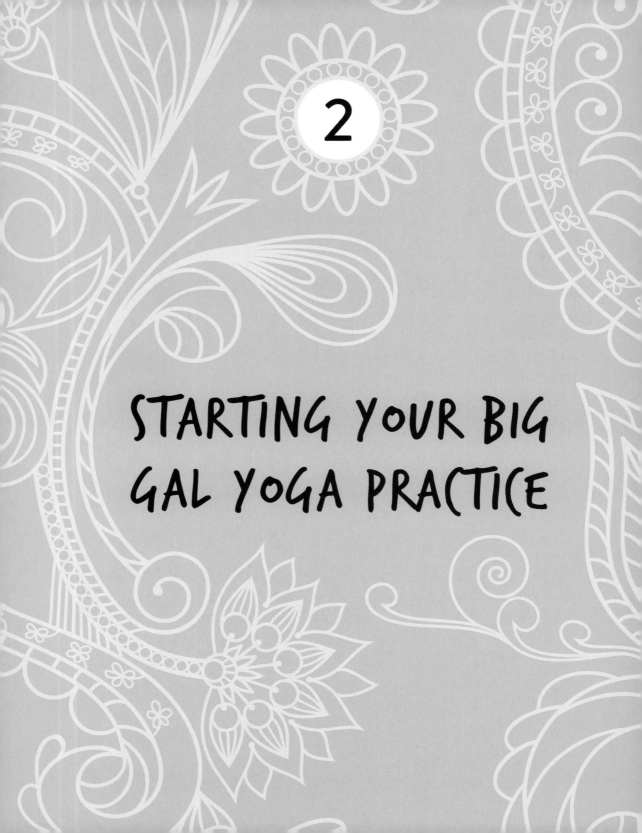

2

STARTING YOUR BIG GAL YOGA PRACTICE

TYPES OF YOGA

The first question many people are faced with when they want to start a yoga practice is what type of yoga to try. All yoga poses, or *asana*, are based on Hatha Yoga. However, there are many different styles of yoga, depending on different gurus or masters that create their own programs. The most widely popular yoga *asana* practice today is a fast-paced yoga practice called Vinyasa. I began in a Hatha Yoga class that included a series of postures that balance each other out just like the sun *ha* and moon *tha* do. The poses work with the breath and balancing the body.

There are dozens of different styles of yoga practices. Each practice is based on the order and repetition of various poses. The differences between the practices involve the choices of poses held, the length of time they are held for, alignment, how to enter the posture, and how to breathe before, during, and afterwards. Some are fast paced with a lot of dynamic energy, and others are restorative, using long static poses.

Some of the practices you'll see offered both in yoga studios and online include:

+ **ASHTANGA:** Ashtanga is considered the mother of all Vinyasa yoga practices: it is physically challenging, focusing on strength, endurance, alignment, breath, and repetition to create purification of the body, mind, and senses. The practice consists of a set of Sun Salutations A and B, a standing sequence, and one of the six series from the primary, intermediate, or advanced series.

+ **BIKRAM:** Known to most as "hot yoga," Bikram yoga is named after its founder, Bikram Choudhury. The practice is taught to his exact specifications: the yoga studio has to be heated to 105 degrees, and the routine is a completely fixed set of twenty-six poses.

+ **IYENGAR:** Named after B. K. S. Iyengar, this is a style of Hatha Yoga that focuses on technique, sequence, and timing. It focuses on holding poses for long periods of time, and how the sequences are put together determine the effect on the body.

+ KUNDALINI: This is a more spiritual practice that works with *kriyas*. It in-volves meditation, dynamic exercises, breathing techniques, and chanting mantras to awaken spiritual energy.

+ POWER: Power Yoga is closely related to the Ashtanga practice and is known as a vigorous, physically challenging, fitness-based style of yoga workout.

+ VINYASA: This is a term that refers to any yoga practice with "flow," where one posture leads into another without stopping. The body and breath flow together from pose to pose in a fast-paced practice.

+ YIN: This is a slower-paced practice, where you hold poses for longer peri-ods of time, 3–5 minutes, to stretch the deep connective tissue. These poses are less strenuous and let you sink into the posture to enhance circulation to the joints, helping with flexibility.

The next issue is deciding where you will practice yoga. There are benefits to all kinds of different practice environments, including doing yoga at home or at a studio.

I've experienced the benefits of both environments, and I encourage you to try both to see what works best for you. After my initial college yoga class, I felt con-fident with my yoga practice, and now I prefer to practice yoga at home in my backyard. Yet when I first started, I enjoyed learning with a big group of people, especially in a big class. Sometimes I'll choose where to do yoga depending on my mood: if I'm feeling too stuck in my own head, I'll go to a class so I can let myself be guided by a teacher. If I want some quiet time to myself, I'll roll out my mat at home.

CREATING A HOME PRACTICE

A home yoga practice is a wonderful thing. We often feel most comfortable in the safety and privacy of our own space. If you choose to do yoga at home you can do it any time of the day or night. It's also a good way to carve out time in your day just for yourself.

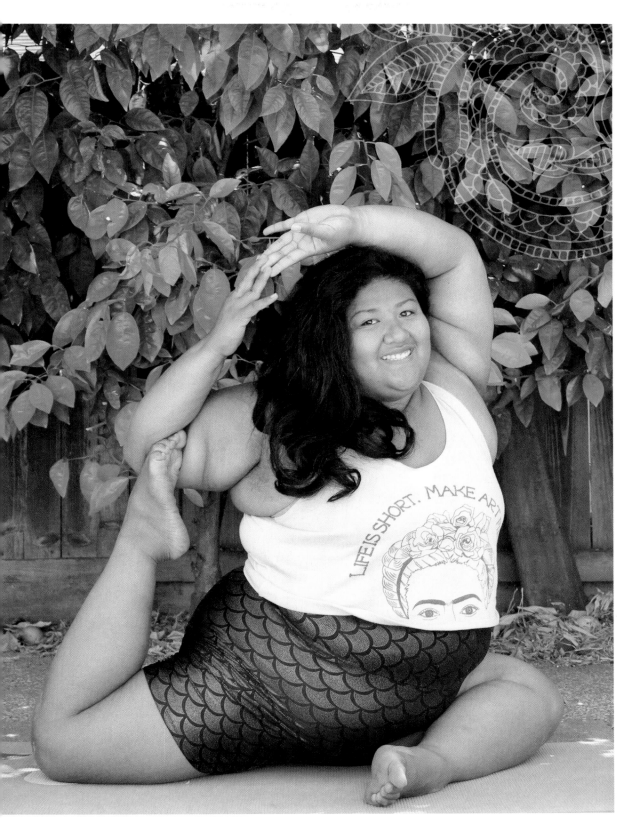

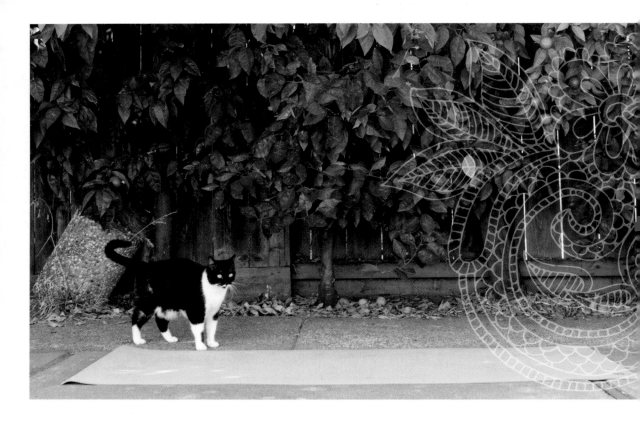

Once I was able to memorize the basic routines from my yoga classes, I began to practice alone at home. For me, there are fewer distractions at home, and I can focus on myself better than I can in a class. When I'm by myself, I can work at my own pace, and focus my practice on whatever I want to, including working on specific areas of my body, and specific poses.

You don't need much room at home, either: just roll out a yoga mat and you're all set. You might want to have access to a clear wall for support, and a chair with a solid back, but that's about it. If there is a mirror in the room, even better, but it's not required. Having a little altar, a nice little space just for you, and focusing on yourself with the music you like, makes for a great retreat. I know that sometimes just having a private spot is a luxury, so pick out a little area for yourself whether it's the corner of a room or a spot in your backyard.

One thing I recommend from time to time for a home yoga practice is access to the camera on a smartphone, tablet, or camera with a timer. When you're doing poses by yourself, even if you have a mirror, it can be difficult to see if you are holding the pose or posture correctly. The photos help me see what I'm doing either correctly or incorrectly and can also let me see my body in different angles. But even more importantly, it can show me how to correct myself before I get hurt from holding a pose incorrectly.

Online Classes and Internet Yoga

The easiest way to do yoga at home is following along with a book, like this one, or with an online class. There are so many types of yoga classes offered, so try a little bit of everything if you can. See what fits you and your personality. Beginner-friendly yoga online classes like Hatha or a Gentle Vinyasa style are great choices to start with.

Online classes can come in handy if you have a very busy life and can't make it to a studio. In this way, even if you have an extra hour before you go to sleep, you can fit in a yoga class. They are also good if you're a little bit nervous about environments where there are other people who you think will be judging you. The truth is, they are probably not thinking about you at all, but I know that a lot of bigger women I've encountered don't want to feel judged in a class.

The first decision you'll have to make is choosing a resource. There are plenty of free, online yoga services, like www.doyogawithme.com and www.freeyoga.tv, or you can check out what's on YouTube. There are more and more yoga teachers posting all types of classes online for you to practice. However, free yoga is limited at times, and the same thing can happen with using DVDs. If you only have access to one routine with no variation it can get boring. However, it's a great way to try something new with little downside.

Monthly online paid services like www.yogaglo.com, www.yogainternational .com, www.myyogaworks.com, www.ekhartyoga.com, www.codyapp.com, or www .gaia.com are definitely a step up in quality. For one monthly fee, they provide continuously updated resources. The cost of a month might be the same as one class at a "brick and mortar" yoga studio, so there is high value. And, there is often lots of variety; not all studios in your area will offer all of the same courses that you can find online. This fact alone will allow you to be exposed to many more different types of yoga, as well as more of the yoga culture. On the other hand, if you aren't looking for variety, but for one routine that you really connect with, online resources mean that you could follow along with your favorite teacher or routine every day, whenever you wanted.

Practicing Yoga Outdoors

I love practicing yoga outdoors because the air filling your lungs can feel so clean and crisp. You feel like your lungs are expanding with so much good oxygen. When I travel to national parks or other spots outdoors, it is a rejuvenating and peaceful feeling to be one with nature. One of my favorite spots to travel to is Joshua Tree National Park, in the desert near Palm Springs. The feeling there is just amazing and rejuvenating.

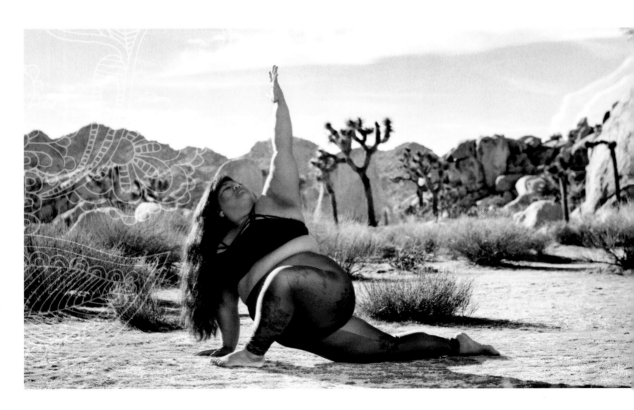

I know that not everyone can live where there is great weather all the time, like it is in California, so if the weather permits in your hometown or when you are on vacation, give outdoor yoga a try.

When I am home, my yoga practice is mainly out in my backyard next to my citrus trees. Granted, I am still in a city with noisy neighbors and low-flying personal planes, but when it's just right, I get my own little slice of peace outdoors.

JOINING A STUDIO

It can also be a lot of fun to dive into the yoga community and practice with a group. Being in an actual yoga studio is a great experience—there is always so much energy in the room. I know for many of us who don't fit the traditional yoga image of a skinny, fit white woman, the idea of unrolling our mats in a class might be daunting. I promise, it will be worth the effort. Get out there and represent!

Some people find the class environment more motivating than practicing at home, especially if they can go with a friend. I tend to go to yoga studios by myself, but I know that for many people, having someone with you helps socially. A studio is all about creating a community. Having somebody that you already know makes people feel comfortable. For instance, my first two students that I had were like twins, and they always showed up together. They felt comfortable because they liked to play off each other and have fun in the class.

Another benefit of live classes is that a teacher will tell you what to do and how you can improve. Even in large classes, the instructor can correct you if your alignment is off and make sure you're not going to hurt yourself. I've met lots of people who have told me that they are scared to sit up front at a yoga studio because they either felt insecure about their level of expertise or were nervous that the teacher would use them in a demonstration. I definitely have a fear of others just staring at me. However, I consciously try to sit in front of the class. The closer I am to the teacher, the more knowledge I receive.

When you are searching for a yoga studio, don't judge a class by its size. The minimum space you will need is just the size of your mat, and the maximum is not much more. I've been to giant yoga classes that have hundreds of people, where

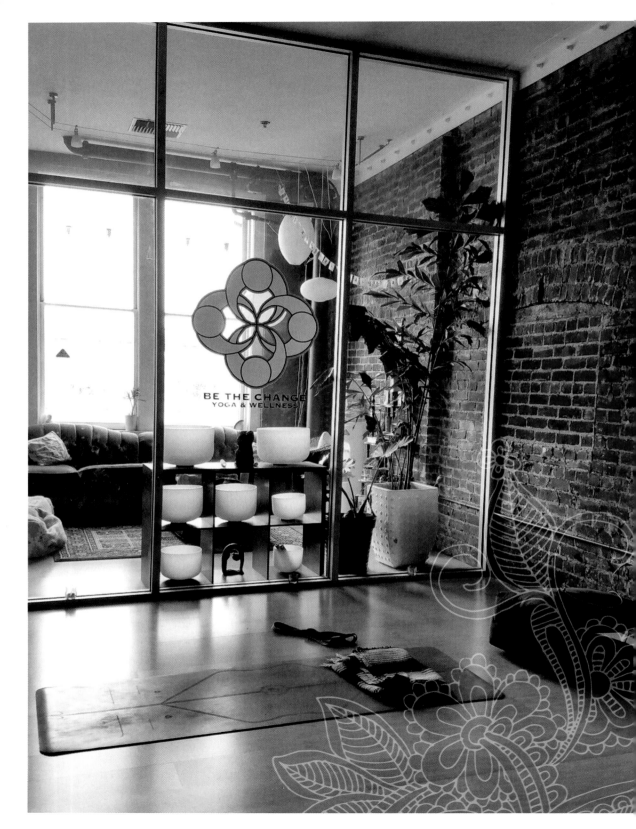

there has been no room for spreading your arms out without touching someone. Rest assured, classes are always set up so that there is more than enough room.

Keep in mind that yoga classes can be expensive. It's a good idea to check out Groupon or LivingSocial for local yoga studio deals. Try out a few different studios and classes to see which one fits you. I've gone to classes thinking, *"This type of practice sounds cool,"* only to find that it totally wasn't for me. It's all about trial and error and finding a good fit for you. The more you try, the more likely it will be that you'll find the one class or teacher that makes you feel the most at ease.

It's also a good idea to try a class a few times before you make a firm decision to not try it again. Don't just judge a class the first time you try it. For instance, during my Hatha Yoga teacher training, I fell in love with Kundalini, and now I want to do Kundalini teacher training. Oddly enough, the class that I thought I would never try again was Kundalini. I took a class at a studio near me and the description sounded interesting, but when I took the class I wasn't connecting to the teacher and the practice. However, at teacher training my teachers presented the practice in a different way, which completely changed my mind about it.

GET IN GEAR: YOGA CLOTHES, PROPS, AND MATS

Regardless of whether you are practicing yoga at home or in a studio, you don't need anything besides determination and positive motivation. However, before you hit the mat and try out your first pose, you might like to gather a few props and pieces of clothing that are best suited to yoga.

Clothes

In terms of clothes, you want to be comfortable, but at the same time, covered for all your angles. I know that some big gals feel a little insecure wearing tight-fitting things. However, baggy clothes don't really work well for yoga because as you bend they will drape down and block your view, a distraction from your practice. I've had the experience in class where I thought I had dressed comfortably, only to find that I was worrying about my clothes and not paying attention to my practice. When it comes to yoga pants, it's important to practice in something that fits well. Being distracted by clothes moving around or rough or rubbing fabric is the worst! Now, it may be that your body isn't going to perfectly fit the shape of any pair of leggings—your body is special and different, and even the most expensive pair may create some rolling at the waist or clinging at the hip. That's okay! Find a pair that feels soft and fits without binding, and the more you wear them, the more they'll adjust to your shape. My first leggings came from Target—they were a nice and cheap $12 pair that, by the way, I still have after all these years! There was nothing fancy about them—they were light and comfortable—but my body was not made for low-waisted leggings. Still, they did their job for me back then.

Today, yoga clothing companies are booming online. There are still fewer options for bigger bodies, but there are more companies starting to extend their sizes. Having all those choices means I can be picky about what I wear—and it's good to be picky. We shouldn't have to compromise! For me, the most important factor for choosing leggings is tummy coverage. I like my tummy to be held in place while I'm moving and bending; that's why I have to make sure I get high-waisted leggings.

In addition to tummy control, there are many factors to consider when buying leggings. Take into account what you like: Do you prefer lighter-weight or thicker fabric? Does it have tummy coverage or booty coverage? Do you prefer cotton or spandex fabric? Do the seams fall comfortably? Try moving, twisting, and stretching in them. Is any part of your body unnecessarily restricted?

I've tried many different brands and can find something good and bad about each different one. Some have awesome prints, better quality of material and stitching, variations of size and fit, and more. Some are big brands; others come from small businesses that can cater to your body size. Here are a few brands you might like to try that cater to a big gal body:

- ✦ Fractal 9
- ✦ Lineagewear
- ✦ A-Bomb Apparel
- ✦ Rainbeau Curves
- ✦ Bombsheller
- ✦ Zions Den Apparel
- ✦ K-Deer
- ✦ Personal Record
- ✦ Lucy Activewear
- ✦ JCPenney Boutique+
- ✦ Torrid

Props

First things first: you don't *need* props. I started my yoga practice without any props. However, props can be beneficial for everyone, and they can be particularly helpful for bigger-bodied yogis. When practicing yoga, it is essential to know your body well—what are its strengths? Its limitations? Where might you need a little more assistance? This is where props come in. Props can remove physical obstacles—as well as mental fears that might hold you back. As you're working to gain more flexibility, props let you complete the poses. We often hold ourselves back from even trying some of the poses. Not being able to complete a pose can be very discouraging. However, just having a simple pair of blocks can help you. Eventually, as you become more flexible, you can move the blocks away, and touch the floor.

When practicing yoga *asana*, it's important to feel comfortable in any position. That means noticing when our bodies are feeling strained or unnecessarily uncomfortable, and we listen to and respect our bodies and what they're telling us. If you feel something is seriously hurting or a position doesn't feel secure, stop and find another approach, possibly by using a prop.

When I first started practicing yoga, I was always trying to prove to myself that I didn't need props. I wanted to rely on my *own* power and strength. I soon found that using props to support my body and my practice didn't mean I wasn't powerful and strong—it simply meant that my body's strength was best put into action with some supportive tools. I can't say this strongly enough: *using props does not mean that you are weak or not doing it the "right way."* It is not worth hurting yourself out of pride or fear of what other people might think.

However, this doesn't mean you need to spend a fortune on props. In fact, you can even make them yourself right at home—I've used everything from stacks of paper for blocks and my phone charger as a strap! There are loads of ways you can improvise. You can use scarves, extra T-shirts, or you can get all DIY and make your own straps out of sewn fabric or crochet. If you would like a block, you can use a stack of heavy books to prop yourself up. If you are old school and still have old VHS tapes lying around, you can tape a couple of them together for a repurposed block. Whether you plan to make, buy, beg, borrow, or repurpose, make it your own, so it works for your budget and body.

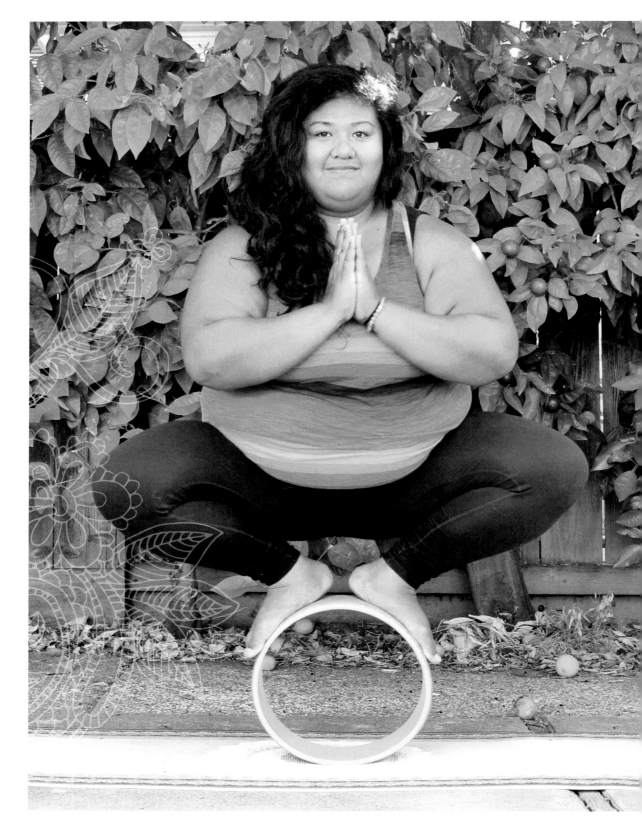

Here are a few items you might like to have nearby when you're practicing yoga. You can purchase all props from companies like Hugger Mugger, JadeYoga, Manduka, Gaiam, Liforme, Infinity Strap, Prana, I Love Gurus, indie small yoga businesses, or www.yogaoutlet.com and www.amazon.com.

BLOCKS

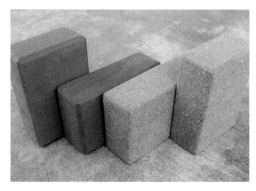

In poses that call for one or both hands to touch the floor, having a block can be a big help. You can place a block in front of you, essentially "raising" the floor so that you can connect your hand(s) to the ground. This helps to keep the body aligned safely in certain poses. Blocks are particularly useful in poses such as a Low Lunge, Forward Fold, or Half Moon.

There are all different types of blocks. There is foam, cork, or wood in different thicknesses and sizes: standard rectangle, rounded, oval, or wedges. Studios often offer foam blocks because they are light and easy to store and keep clean. I prefer cork blocks because they are made from sustainable resources, are resistant to sweat so you won't slip, and are heavier so they don't easily move around.

STRAPS

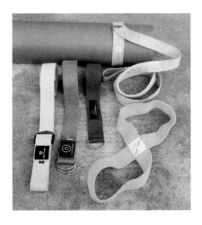

Straps look like a belt. They can range from 4 feet to 8 feet and are made of cotton or hemp. There are also straps made from a stretchy material that allow you to have more wiggle room in the pose, unlike the cotton ones, which are static. Straps can be used as an "extending arm," usually when a pose calls for a connection of the hand and foot. In these poses—such as Dancer Pose, Bow Pose, and Supine Spinal Twist—it can be difficult to fully grab your foot with your hand. Looping your foot with a strap offers you a little more extension. You may find you want to use a strap every time you practice, or you may use it until a stretch becomes more comfortable, deeper, and then the strap is no longer needed.

Larger bodies do not need larger straps. The length of your strap just depends on your level of flexibility. Some people are naturally flexible even if they are big. Then there are other people who have tighter hips or muscles. Those are the ones that need the longer straps.

BOLSTERS

Bolsters are rectangular, round, or oblong cushions that come in a variety of sizes. They are used for propping up parts of your body when you are practicing meditative or restorative poses. My own favorite way of using a bolster is to place its end at the base of my spine while sitting in a Bound Angle Pose, then relaxing over it to open up my heart and chest (you'll learn more about this on page 183). The bolster is also great for relieving back pain while lying in Savasana—the final relaxation pose.

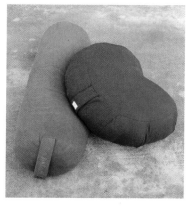

No matter how much I practice, I still get twinges of lower back pain while lying flat on my back, so I often place a bolster underneath my knees to relieve pain or pressure. Bolsters can also be used to support your body if you are going to sit for long periods during meditation.

BLANKETS

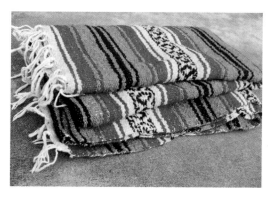

Blankets used for yoga are usually made of thick cotton. They can be folded into many different shapes and then used for support. Rolling a blanket as a bolster is great because you can adjust the height depending on how you roll it. When I am in a cross-legged position or a seated pose for a long time, I like to sit on a folded blanket to relieve pressure on my sit bones. I fold it a couple inches thick, so it supports the base of my spine, elevating my hips. A blanket can also be used for a bit of cushion support if you are on your hands and knees on the mat. Place it under your wrists to alleviate wrist pain, or under your knees to cushion direct contact to the mat. You can also roll it up into a long tube to use as a strap.

CHAIR

Using a chair is a great way to practice up off the floor. There are even yoga classes that use the chair for the whole class. The chair offers modified versions of poses so that you can work towards more flexibility. It is a way to practice the motions of a pose higher up, similar to using blocks, where you want a hand-to-floor connection for stability and balance, but just with more height. Practicing poses with the chair can work for poses like Cat/ Cow Pose, Extended Triangle, or Wheel Pose.

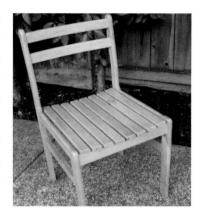

YOGA WHEEL

The yoga wheel is a circular device that is used for support during a back-bend posture. Yoga wheels are relatively new to the scene and are considered a luxury item. They typically come in three diameter sizes: 10, 12, and 15 inches, and all are roughly 4 inches wide. They can be wooden or made from PVC piping and can have

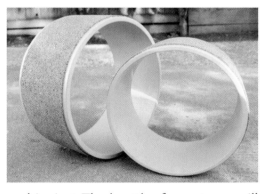

foam or cork on the outside for grip or cushioning. The length of your torso will determine which size you should get. I am short and have a short torso, so the 10 inch works best for me.

Yoga wheels support you as you increase your range of movement and allow you to try out poses that may seem far out of reach. In some ways, they have the same uses and extending quality of a block, but they are not as static because they move around with you. They are definitely amazing for opening up your back—even just lying over one and rolling back and forth is a great way to massage the spine while bending the back at the same time.

HAND TOWELS

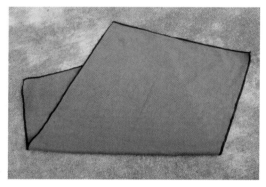

Have a small towel nearby when you're practicing yoga—you'll be glad it's there! You're likely to get sweaty, and if you don't have a clean cloth in arm's reach, you'll wind up like me, using the hem of your shirt to wipe away the sweat. It's better to grab a hand towel quickly and wipe the sweat away so you can get back to concentrating on your practice. There are specific microfiber yoga towels that absorb more sweat, or you can use a regular cotton hand towel.

Yoga Mats

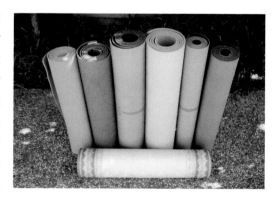

Having a yoga mat is great, but it's totally not essential—you can easily practice on the floor, on a towel, or on a blanket. Mats come in a variety of colors, materials, and prices. You don't have to spend a fortune to get a good mat, but I'll admit that the more expensive ones do offer nice features! As a beginner, low-cost mats around

$20 can do the job. Once you get deeper into your yoga practice, if you want more out of your mat, a nice-quality mat is a good investment.

Mats can be made from lots of different types of materials, including PVC, natural tree rubber, and cork, each of which offers different surface feels. They can also range in thickness: thin ones are great for easy traveling, while thicker ones supply more cushioning. Right now I'm favoring the ones made from natural rubber. Still, the one that works best for you may be a basic $20 mat, so give a simple one a try before splurging.

SIMPLE DIY MAT CLEANER

Because you'll be sweating a lot, you need to keep your mat clean. There are a lot of mat sprays that the big yoga brands sell, or you can make your own with essential oils, distilled water, and witch hazel or vinegar. You can also clean your mat with a natural or regular antibacterial wipe.

Combine the following in an 8-ounce spray bottle:

+ 1½ ounces witch hazel or vinegar
+ 6 ounces distilled water
+ 2–4 drops tea tree essential oil
+ 1–3 drops lavender essential oil

Shake the bottle to mix ingredients, and spray a light layer over your mat, wiping it off with a paper or cotton towel.

Mats are usually recommended for yoga because they can be both cushiony and grippy. Bigger gals might think they want a lot more cushion, like the extra-thick exercise mats, but I'd advise against it. Softer mats are made from plastic materials that, while cushiony, can tend to make you slip, as well as being too soft to move around on more easily. If it can hold you in a Downward Dog without slipping, you're good. Also, if a mat is too cushiony it can make you sink into it, forcing your body out of alignment. If you want site-specific spots for cushioning, use other props like blankets in the areas you need it. Look for a mat that seems sticky to the touch, is firm, and at the max one-quarter inch thick.

Here are a few mat brands you might like to consider:

JADE—Jade mats from JadeYoga usually run around $70, but you can find good sales from time to time. I was lucky to find a $20 Jade mat at an REI gear sale when I got my first one. This was a great deal, especially considering the quality of the mat: it is made with an eco-friendly rubber that makes for a good grip. If you can tolerate the smell of natural rubber, this is a great mat to use. Avoid storing in direct sunlight (as well as practicing for long periods outdoors) because it will ruin the stickiness of the rubber.

MANDUKA—I've had two Manduka mats: the eKO SuperLite Travel Mat ($42) and the PRO yoga mat ($110). The travel mat has a very good grip, and even though it lacks thickness, it is great for traveling because it's lightweight and foldable. Sometimes I liked to place it on a thicker mat for better cushion and grip. The PRO mat, on the other hand, is a big fella! It's definitely one of those mats that is a "home mat," which means it's not great for traveling because it is dense and heavy. It's not one of my preferred mats.

LIFORME—I've seen many of the famous yoga practitioners using this mat. I finally got the chance to try one out for myself and see what the rage was, and now I understand. This is hands down an incredible mat! The grip is spot on; it's eco-friendly, doesn't have a weird smell, comes with a nice carrying case, is a good weight (not too heavy) for easy transportation, absorbs oil and moisture, is easy to

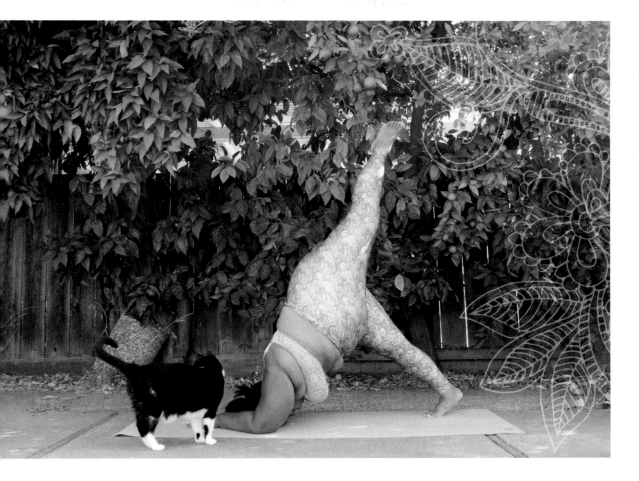

clean—it's a hit! They keep it simple with four bold colors and lines etched into the mat that are great for alignment. The only downside to this mat is the price: at $140 it's definitely high end. For that reason, it may not be a great choice as a starter mat, but as you get more serious about practicing yoga, it's a great investment in your practice considering the amazing quality.

GAIAM—A Gaiam mat was the first mat I ever bought. I recently have tried the Gaiam Studio Select Dry-Grip mat. This mat reminds me of Liforme because of the top surface grip (though it's still not as sticky as the Liforme) and is sold at a much more affordable price ($60–$70). The difference is that it is not made of natural rubber. It is a nice mat if you want to upgrade to a better-quality mat and are okay with a little bit of PVC smell. Gaiam also sells a large array of low-priced mats, one of which you might want to try out. My first mat was a Gaiam mat for $20, and it served me well at beginning of my practice.

There are definitely high-priced yoga mats out there that you can find great deals on at places like www.yogaoutlet.com or www.amazon.com. I have found great deals from REI at used gear sales, and their clearance is great. On top of that, you can purchase the mat, and if it doesn't work for your body, you may return it within a year. Most places don't let you return anything if it's used!

GET READY TO BEGIN: FINDING YOUR MOTIVATION

Finding, and then maintaining, a sense of motivation can be one of the hardest steps to starting anything new—even a yoga practice that is guaranteed to enrich your physical health, mental state, and spirit.

Working on this book took a lot of my mat time because I knew I had to get this out for you guys! But after sitting here crunched up, typing for hours, I'm more motivated than ever to get back to my practice. Taking classes again will help to get some energy moving through my body and open up the tight parts that have gotten stiff from sitting all day; it will allow me to feel like myself again.

Many of us use the new year to start challenging ourselves to change something that we've struggled with in the past, whether it's losing weight, letting go of toxic individuals or a bad habit, trying new things, or meeting new people. I've tried making New Year's resolutions for many years and have failed every time. I finally realized that a new year alone wasn't offering me enough motivation to change my behavior: it's just a totally arbitrary date on the calendar, really no different than any other. I also realized that I wasn't really committed to making those resolutions, and I didn't enjoy the process of what I thought I had to do in order to keep them. I learned that if you don't enjoy what you do you'll never get motivated.

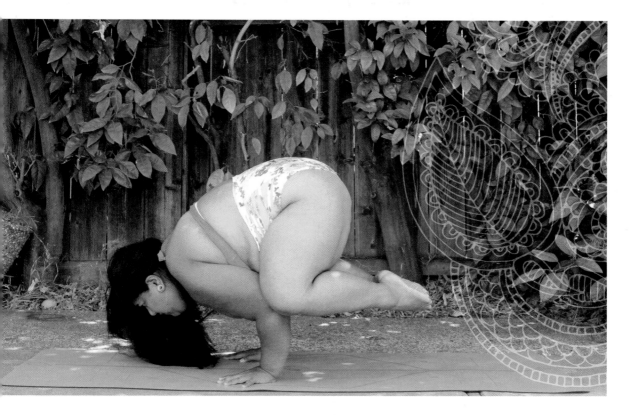

Motivation Tips

I still go through periods where I gain and then lose motivation, which is definitely normal but can be frustrating at times. Even now that I've made yoga my full-time occupation, it is sometimes hard for me to motivate myself to get on my mat.

I've found that there is no single method for keeping yourself connected to a yoga practice, but I do have a couple of suggestions. First, as I mentioned before, I was fortunate to learn yoga in an academic setting that required me to go to yoga class two times a week. This helped me to develop a steady home practice afterwards. It's definitely tricky for people starting out to keep up a regular schedule because our lives are so busy with work, family, and social obligations, not to mention the cost and availability of classes that fit your needs. Sometimes staying motivated can be as simple as forcing yourself to set aside a small amount of time dedicated to you and your practice. Even 10–30 minutes, one to three times a week, is a good amount of time to start, focus, and learn something new.

Find others to motivate and inspire you. Social media is great for that. When I started there was a very limited number of plus-size yogis across any media. I found them mainly at niche websites, and these sites weren't interactive like Instagram, Tumblr, Twitter, or Facebook. Pioneers like Amber Karnes and Dianne Bondy were kicking off the body positive yoga movement, and I looked to them as great role models. I also took inspiration from other beautiful yogis who didn't look like me. I didn't aspire to look like them size-wise, but to learn from their practices in order to further my own. I drew motivation from yoga challenges hosted by fellow Tumblr and Instagram yogis. Go online and find the people who motivate you to be your best.

"Most people can motivate themselves to do things simply by knowing that those things need to be done. But not me. For me, motivation is this horrible, scary game where I try to make myself do something while I actively avoid doing it. If I win, I have to do something I don't want to do. If I lose, I'm one step closer to ruining my entire life. And I never know whether I'm going to win or lose until the last second."

—ALLIE BROSH,
HYPERBOLE AND A HALF

Set goals that are manageable. Doing a pose a day as a challenge helped get me on my mat even if it was just for that one pose. Once I was there, I usually stayed on my mat to practice more.

Lastly, be kind to yourself. Don't get me wrong—being active is vital and beneficial to your well-being, but you don't need to beat yourself up if you skip a day, or if you don't reach a certain goal. Life is a process of constant change—one year we can have more free time, and the next year we are strapped with unexpected obligations. We're not machines—schedules change, shit happens, and life gets in the way. We all have complicated lives. If you find you're off course, get back on schedule when you can, and appreciate all parts of the journey.

OPENING YOUR PRACTICE: SANTOSHA

Whenever I teach a beginner yoga class, I start off chanting the word *santosha*. This is one of the *niyamas*, positive observances, of the eight limbs of yoga. *Santosha* means "contentment." We often want to already be "perfect" in every part of our life, including our yoga practice. We want to already be flexible or strong before we have even gotten a chance to start; we want to be just like someone we've seen in class, on a website, or in a video. *Santosha* means that you are instead finding contentment in your own physical and mental abilities, in the moment, and accepting yourself as you are now.

If you're starting something new, like this yoga challenge, and you're getting discouraged because you can't be perfect, using the word *santosha* takes some of the pressure off. Remember, yoga can feel differently to you every day; that's why it's called a practice. There is no perfection. Over time, your yoga abilities will change, and you'll eventually see progress. You just have to give yourself time and be kind to yourself.

You can make *santosha* part of your vocabulary or daily mind-set during the following challenge, or for any other yoga practice. Sit down on the mat. Take a few breaths. Close your eyes. Say *santosha* aloud three times. Or, chant it to yourself whenever you need to be reminded that there is contentment within imperfection.

PRANAYAMA: YOGA BREATHING

Pranayama means "control of the breath." The breath is *prana*, your life force. Having control of your breath promotes concentration and improves vitality while allowing oxygen to flow through the cells within the body. This is essential for being conscious of the mind-body connection during your yoga practice. It can help you monitor your mood, giving you a sense of calmness and reducing stress and anxiety.

While breathing is an involuntary action, happening automatically without thought, there are actually different ways to breathe. When we apply some thought to the way we breathe we can make the most of the energy we are generating. By staying mindfully aware of breathing and doing it well, you can set the right rhythm of inhalations and exhalations, which promotes calm and alleviates negativity, creating a more fulfilling time spent on the mat.

BENEFITS OF PRANAYAMA

+ Circulates oxygen through the bloodstream
+ Relieves tension in the body
+ Moves energy throughout the body
+ Creates awareness of presence
+ Helps to regulate blood pressure when agitated or stressed
+ Calms the mind

The point of the following breathing exercises is to expand your lungs. Most people don't inhale deeply all the time, and usually take quick, short breaths. Breathing poorly can trigger a panicked response from the body, increasing anxiety and compromising your health. The yoga breathing techniques teach you to expand the lungs and be able to take in more oxygen, because the more oxygen you're able to inhale, the better your body feels.

Ujjayi Breath

The most common controlled breath used in a class is called *ujjayi* (pronounced *oo-jah-ee*). During the yoga challenge, or whenever you are taking a yoga class or practicing yoga on your own, use this breathing technique as you flow from pose to pose. It will help you find a rhythm of inhales and exhales.

Find a nice, comfortable, seated position. You can use props, like a bolster or blanket. You can be cross-legged on the floor, on a chair, or however you feel most comfortable. Then, slowly close the eyes, placing the hands onto the knees. Don't rush through the breathing practice.

To begin, imagine that there is a glass window or mirror in front of you. Open your mouth breathing out to pretend to slowly fog up the window. As you do this, slightly constrict the back of your throat. As you inhale and exhale, try to maintain that constriction in the throat. Then, try the exact same process ("fogging up the window") with your mouth closed, keeping that constriction in the back of your throat as you inhale and exhale. The *ujjayi* breath should sound like an ocean breeze, or the Darth Vader breath, as you breathe in and out through your nose. Sometimes you're the only one who can hear it, or it can be loud if you prefer.

COUNTING YOUR BREATH TECHNIQUE

The best way to train your *ujjayi* breath is by controlling your breathing by counting your inhalations, holds, and exhalations. Over time, this will slowly expand your lungs and your ability to take in deeper and longer breaths.

Start with a four-part breathing exercise:

+ Establish a calm normal *ujjayi* breath.

+ Taking four slow counts, exhale all of the air in your lungs starting at the bottom of the lungs, closest to your stomach, and exhaling all the air up through your chest, until it feels as though there is no more air in the lungs.

+ Once the lungs are empty, hold the exhaled breath for another four counts.

+ Slowly and calmly inhale, counting to four while expanding the lungs. With awareness of your breath, fill the lungs, starting at the top of the chest and filling the lungs all the way down towards the stomach to the count of four.

+ Hold the air in the lungs as you slowly count to four. Pay attention to the sensation, how it feels to have all that air occupy your lungs.

+ Once you are done holding, repeat the first step by steadily exhaling, starting at the bottom of the lungs and emptying all the breath out of your chest while counting to four.

+ You can keep practicing with the four count, or expand to a five or eight count, or to however long feels good to you.

Other Breathing Techniques

There are other yoga breathing techniques you might want to try. For example, you can isolate your breath to specific parts of your body. These techniques allow you to have even more control of your breath. You will be shifting your awareness to a specific area of the body, breathing to the belly, back, or sides. Remember, don't rush through the breathing practice.

BELLY BREATHING

One technique is called belly breathing. Here you focus on the rise and fall of the belly as you inhale and exhale.

+ Begin by lying on your back, finding a comfortable position. Place a bolster, pillow, or rolled-up blanket under the knees. Close the eyes and begin breathing with a steady breath.

+ As you inhale, focus on your belly and let it expand, and fill it completely with air. The belly then drops down as your exhale.

+ Repeat this belly breathing for 5 minutes, keeping your awareness on that specific area. I find it helpful to put my hands on my belly as I'm breathing, so I can feel how my belly changes with each inhalation and exhalation.

BACK BREATHING

I learned back breathing during my teacher training, taught by Rama Joyti Vernon, and it is a very beneficial technique. It is a way to focus the breath through the back as well as learn to lengthen the spine. This can be practiced in Cat Pose (page 79).

+ Start by coming onto the hands and knees on your mat. The wrists are placed underneath the shoulders, the knees under the hips, and the back flat. If you have a hard time staying on the wrists for a long period of time, place a blanket under only the heel of the hand or drop down to the forearms. If being on the floor is difficult, you can still practice this using a chair (see page 79 for more details).

+ Begin with your natural breath and then start your *ujjayi* breath.

+ On your next inhale, round the back, tucking the tailbone in, and drawing your chin to your chest. Bring your awareness and focus to the spot on the back behind your heart to expand the lungs in that area.

+ As you exhale, flatten the back, creating a pull forward. Straighten the back, pulling forward at the crown of the head, lengthening your vertebrae as you pull back with your hips.

+ Repeat, each time breathing and expanding the lungs at the point behind the heart as you round the back, and exhale out the crown, lengthening the spine. Practice this for 1–3 minutes at a slow and steady pace, creating awareness of the expansion of the breath on your back.

ALTERNATE NOSTRIL (*NADI SHODHANA*)

This breathing exercise is a way of clearing out the channels of air circulation. The fingers alternate back and forth opening and closing the right and left side of the nostrils so we are able to focus on each side. It is a great practice for quieting the mind before a meditation practice, or before a public speaking event to help reduce stress and anxiety.

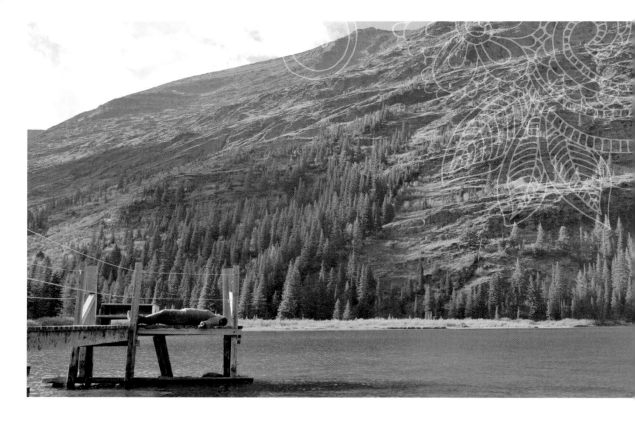

+ Begin in a comfortable seated position with or without props. Sit upright with the spine lengthened and eyes closed. Don't rush through the breathing practice.

+ Place the left hand comfortably down on the left knee or lap. Bring the right hand up, hovering in front of the face. Place your middle and pointer finger between the eyebrows. This will help keep your hand steady as you will be actively using both the thumb and ring finger throughout the exercise.

+ Start by inhaling and exhaling through both nostrils. Before the next inhale, place the thumb on the right nostril to inhale only through the left nostril. As you inhale, slowly fill the lungs all the way up.

+ Hold the breath; lift the thumb off the right nostril to place the ring finger on top of the left nostril, exhaling through the right nostril. Then inhale through the right nostril.

+ Lift the ring finger up to place the thumb on the right nostril, exhaling through the left nostril, and then inhaling through the left nostril.

+ Repeat on each side, remembering to inhale and exhale on each side before switching. Practice 5–30 rounds of this alternate nostril breathing.

+ After your rounds, come back to a natural breath, and take a moment to feel the difference within the body and lungs.

FOCAL POINT (*DRISHTI*)

Drishti is a single-point focusing technique that is used to still the mind. This helps the mind to concentrate and focus as the body is being engaged. In meditation the focal point can be internal, closing the eyes, gazing at the center of the forehead (the Third Eye Chakra), or it can be external, gazing at a candle or symbol on the wall. The focal point in yoga postures is meant to create focus of the mind so the body can be still and engaged into the pose. This is very helpful for balancing poses. Our bodies are wiggling around as they are being accustomed to new poses, and we can tend to overthink and fall out of the pose. Taking a moment to gaze off into the distance at your focal point helps discourage the mind from overthinking, and it will allow the body to move into the position with more ease. So to find your *drishti*, find a spot at eye level off into the distance or on the wall, gazing softly. The eyes want to be calm and relaxed. As your eyes physically gaze at the point, this will refocus the mind inward to help the body remain calm as you enter a posture. Stay on that focal point throughout the posture, or there might be a few different *drishti* as you move around.

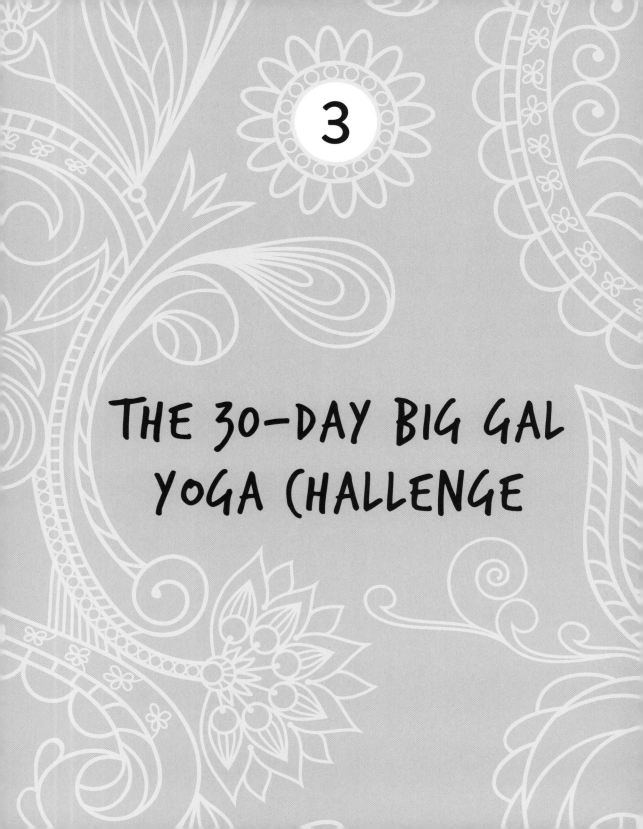

3

THE 30-DAY BIG GAL YOGA CHALLENGE

THE BIG GAL YOGA CHALLENGE

Now you're ready to take on my 30-day yoga challenge. The challenge is meant to offer you a fundamental and accessible way to start your own yoga practice without stressing you out about how to fit one more thing into your busy schedule. We all have time to do one pose a day, right? Later in the month, as you get into the groove, you'll string together some of the poses to create a yoga flow. At the end of the challenge, you'll have completed an entire yoga routine that you can continue to do in sequence.

Follow the instructions as they are written for each day. They will include how to breathe during the pose and how long to hold the pose. The poses will get progressively more difficult as the month goes on, but don't worry, you'll be able to follow along with ease.

Over the next thirty days, each time you practice a pose, post a photo of yourself on your Instagram or Facebook accounts, tag me @BigGalYoga, and add the hashtag #BGYogatoEmpower so I can follow along on your journey. If posting images of yourself is still a new self-practice, don't worry, there is no pressure to post! Just practice by yourself, and I hope you enjoy the challenge!

So grab your mat, and let's get going. Start by thinking about *santosha*, and just have fun.

DAY I

WARM-UPS

Before starting any yoga practice, it is a good idea to warm up the body so that the muscles and joints are stretched, loose, and ready to move into the different yoga poses. Many of these warm-ups can be practiced sitting down on your mat in a neutral cross-legged position, on a chair, or standing. If you're sitting on the floor you can support yourself with a rolled-up blanket or bolster at the base of the spine. Find a comfortable position and get ready for your practice!

WRISTS—WRIST ROTATIONS AND FINGERTIP PRESS:

These exercises help strengthen the wrists. They are great preparation for poses that involve supporting your weight on your hands.

Figure 8—Bring your hands in front of you at chest height, interlacing your fingers so your knuckles are facing away from you with the palms together. Lead with your middle knuckle, drawing a figure 8. This should activate the muscles and joints in the hands and wrists. Make the figure 8 in one direction for 30 seconds, and then reverse the figure 8 to go in the opposite direction again for another 30 seconds. You should feel a pleasant stretch in your wrists, forearms, and knuckles.

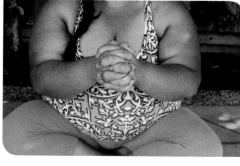
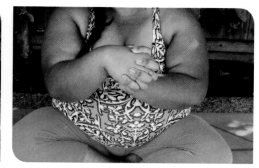

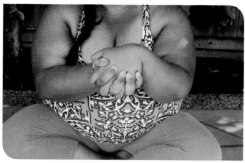
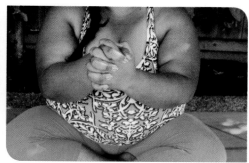

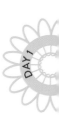

Fingertip press—Release your hands and bring your elbows up to chest height, forearms parallel to the floor. Spread your fingers wide, and touch your fingertips together creating a tent-like shape. Press your fingertips together with even pressure holding for 5 seconds, and then release the pressure for a couple seconds. Repeat for 45 seconds, pressing the fingers for 5 seconds, releasing for a couple seconds, and again pressing the fingertips together.

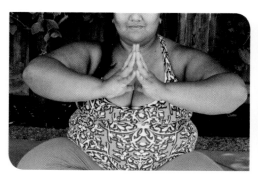
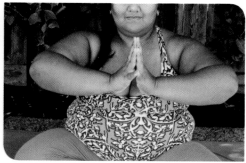

NECK—SIDE TO SIDE, TURNS, FORWARD AND BACK, FOUR-POINT STRETCH:

Throughout our yoga practice, we need to stay aware of the neck. The neck is so important because it connects the head to the rest of the body through the spine. If we overstress our necks, it can cause problems throughout the whole body. Take the time to give your neck some care and attention by stretching it out on all four sides.

Begin with your neck in a neutral and upright position, and then tilt your head to the right side, dropping your ear towards your right shoulder. Feel the muscles along the left side of your neck stretch. Bring your head back to neutral, then repeat, dropping your left ear to your left shoulder and feeling the muscles on the right of the neck stretch. Continue to repeat this stretch, alternating left and right, for 30 seconds. Go at a slow pace and take time to enjoy the stretching sensations.

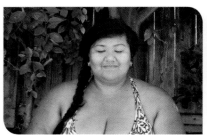 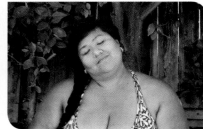 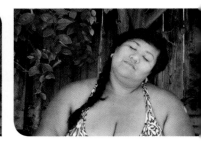

Another side-to-side stretch is neck turns. Begin with the head in a neutral upright position. Turn the head to face towards the right, feeling the neck muscles along the throat stretch. Then turn to face the left, feeling the neck muscles on the right stretch. Go at a slow steady pace for 30 seconds looking right and left. If you want to connect the breath with the movement, inhale as you face right and exhale as you face left.

Next, drop the head back, opening up the throat muscles. Then, moving slowly through the neutral upright position, drop your chin to your chest. You should feel a great stretch down your neck and into your back. Alternate stretching backward and forward for 30 seconds.

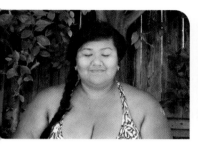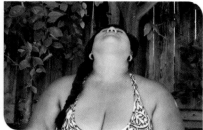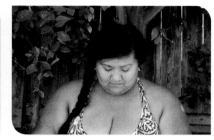

Lastly, going in a clockwise motion, tilt the head to the right, drop the head back, tilt the head to the left, and bring the chin to the chest. Rotate the head for 30 seconds clockwise, and then go in a counterclockwise motion for another 30 seconds.

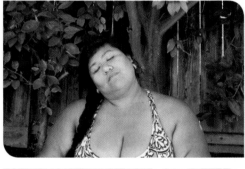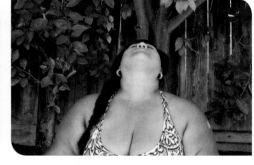

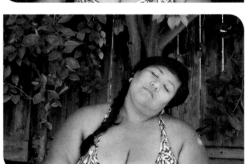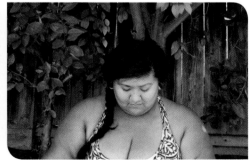

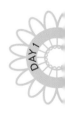

SIDES—SIDE STRETCH AND WAIST ROTATION:

During our practice, the muscles in our torso are always moving and stretching. It's important to get them warmed up so we don't overstress our bodies. These stretches can be performed sitting in a cross-legged position, sitting in a chair, or standing. Choose whatever feels most comfortable.

Begin in a neutral starting position. Inhale and reach both arms up overhead. Exhale and drop your right hand down to floor or right hip by your side. Reach your left hand up and over towards the right side while lengthening your body and neck in the same direction. Hold for 10 seconds.

Inhale; bring your body and right arm back up to a central position. Exhale and drop your left hand down to the floor or left hip by your side. Reach your right hand up and over to the left side, lengthening your body and neck in the same direction. Hold for 10 seconds and feel the muscles on the right side of the body open up. Repeat again on both sides, two more times.

For the seated position, inhale and return to the central position with both arms up. Exhale and twist your torso to the right. Place your left hand on your right knee (use your arms for leverage in the twist) and your right hand on the floor behind your back. Gaze all the way over your right shoulder to get the most from the twist. Hold for 10 seconds. Inhale and reach your arms up, releasing the twist and facing forward. Exhale; drop your right hand down to the left knee and your left hand behind your back. Feel the twist in your torso, and gaze over your left shoulder. Hold for 10 seconds.

If you are in the standing position, take a wider stance with the feet 2 feet apart. Inhale, arms up parallel to the floor, and exhale twisting to the right side. Place the left hand on the right shoulder, and place the right hand on the lower back. Gaze over to the right twisting the torso. Inhale, raising the arms parallel to the floor, and exhale twisting to left side. Right hand on the left shoulder and left hand on the lower back as you twist and gaze over to the left side. Repeat on both sides continuously for 1 minute.

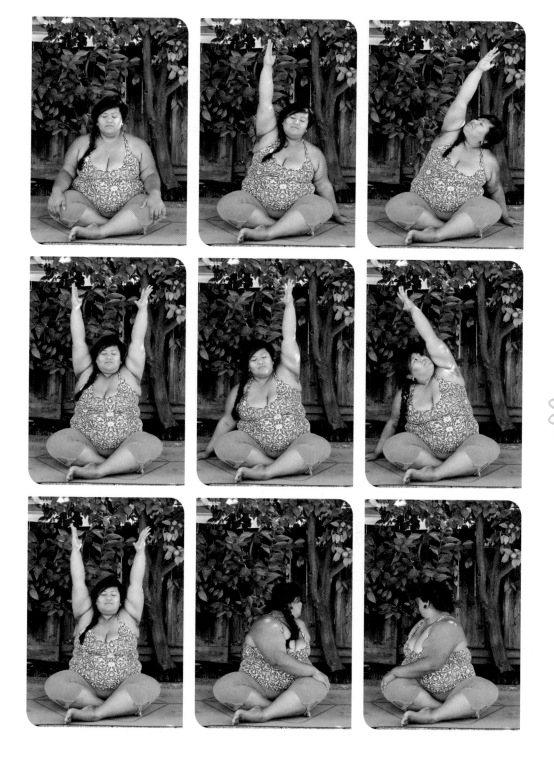

DAY 1

SHOULDERS—SHOULDER ROTATION:

It may not seem like it, but our shoulders do a lot of work during the day, so it's good to give them a little TLC by rotating the joints and stretching the muscles. If you feel like your shoulders are looking a little hunched, this is also great for loosening them up and improving your posture.

Place your hands onto their respective shoulders with the four fingers in front and the thumbs behind. Raise your elbows so your upper arms are parallel to the floor. Start making a circle motion with your elbows. First, forward for about 30 seconds, and then backward for another 30 seconds.

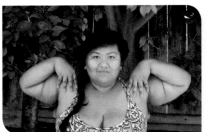 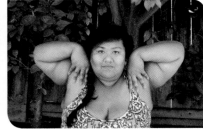 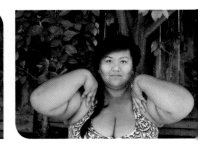

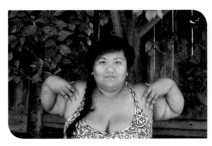 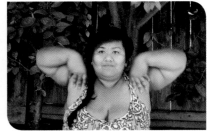

LEGS—LEG LIFTS AND LEGS UP THE WALL:

As hard as we work our arms, our legs are often working even harder. They get us from place to place as we rush around and can feel quite achy by the end of the day. And not working our legs enough can be just as bad—if you sit at a desk all day, you might suffer from poor circulation. A good way to build some fire in your core and strengthen your legs is by doing leg lifts to get the blood flowing through your lower body.

Begin by lying on the floor on your back. If you are having any lower back problems at the moment, place a folded blanket at your sacrum, which is located just above the buttocks. This will help protect the lower back as you lift your legs. Inhale, and raise your straight right leg as close to vertical as you can, then exhale as you drop your leg back down. Next, inhale, raising the left leg up as close to vertical as you can, then exhale as you drop your leg back down. Repeat these alternate leg lifts for 1–2 minutes. Last, inhale and raise both legs up at the same time, then exhale, dropping them back down. Repeat this motion for 30 seconds to 1 minute. You should be feeling a good burn by the end!

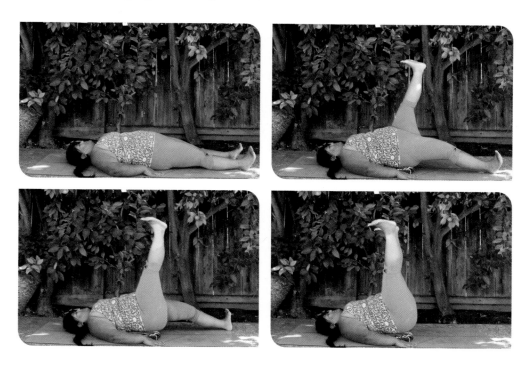

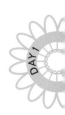

If you have tired legs or feet at the end of the day, a nice way to rest your legs is to bring them up the wall. Even though the position is restorative, you are still stretching the back of the legs, torso, and neck, which helps regulate blood flow through your body. Sit on the floor with your right hip on the wall, and your legs out in front of you. Drop to your left side, and bring your butt as close as you can to the wall. Swing your legs up the wall as you roll onto your back. Your heels should end up on the wall with your feet flexed. Stay here for about 1–2 minutes, maybe also using your belly breathing to keep awareness in the posture. Then swing the legs to the side, pushing yourself back up to an upright position.

ANKLES—ANKLE ROTATION AND FEET FLEX:

Our ankles and feet support our whole body, so they need lots of care. Warming up the ankle joints and feet promotes circulation to prevent your feet from falling asleep. This is a great little stretch that can be done anywhere, anytime.

Begin by sitting on the floor or on a chair with your legs out in front of you (you can use a folded blanket to prop yourself up if needed). Rotate both ankles, drawing circles with your toes, for 30 seconds. Then rotate your ankles in the opposite direction for another 30 seconds. Last, point your toes forward, stretching the tops of the feet, then flex the feet by pointing the toes back towards your body. Repeat this motion for 30 seconds.

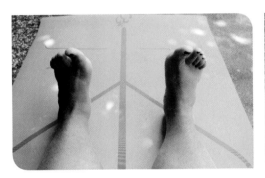 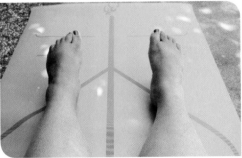

All of these warm-ups can be done before each pose you practice every day of the challenge. It is a good way to get the blood circulating through the body before jumping into the pose!

Now we are all ready to start our yoga practice!

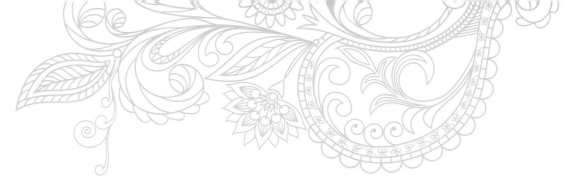

DAY 2

CAT POSE AND COW POSE

(Marjaryasana and Bitilasana)

ABOUT THE POSE:

Cat/Cow is a gentle flow that energizes the body with its grounding position. This pose activates the core, while giving a gentle backbend, and connects your breath with your movement as you arch and round your back like a cat, and drop the belly down like a cow.

BODY BENEFITS:

The flow between the two poses warms up the body, creating flexibility in the spine. This flow opens the chest and stretches the muscles in the neck, back, and torso, while also strengthening the abdominal muscles.

PROPS:

Traditionally Cat/Cow is practiced on the floor with your hands and knees supporting your weight. For some people the pressure on the wrists and knees can be uncomfortable. To help with this you can place a folded blanket under your knees to act as cushioning, and another directly under the wrists to tilt the hands at an angle, creating less pressure on the wrists. If getting up and down from a low hands-and-knees position is difficult, try placing a chair in front of you and resting your hands on the seat with your feet placed firmly on the ground. If it feels like there is too much pressure on your wrists, you can drop down onto your forearms. Keep your elbows aligned underneath your shoulders with your fingers pointing forward. This should relieve any wrist discomfort while still allowing you to go through the motions of the Cat/Cow flow.

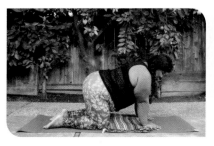 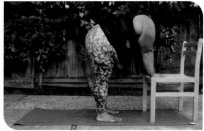 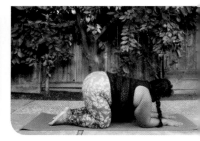

GET IN POSITION:

If you are doing the flow on your hands and knees, align your knees directly under your hips. If you are standing, place your feet hip-width apart. Next, place your hands on the mat or chair, shoulder-width apart and aligned underneath the shoulders. Spread your fingers wide. Keep your back and neck flat and parallel to the floor.

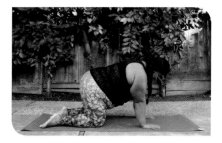

WHEN YOU ARE READY:

Inhale into Cat Pose: Round the back by lifting the center of your back up, tuck in your tailbone, and draw the chin into the chest between the shoulders. Exhale into Cow Pose: Drop your belly down towards the mat, slightly arching the back. Lift the crown of the head and shift the gaze forward. To come out of the pose, bring your body back to a neutral position on all fours. Sit your butt back onto your heels and bring your upper body into an upright position. If you are in a standing position, lift your hands up from the chair, standing upright.

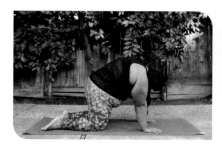 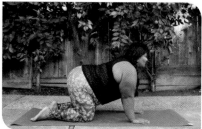

HOW LONG:

Repeat Cat and Cow Poses, staying mindful of your breath throughout. Keep the breath steady, inhaling and exhaling deep with your *ujjayi* breathe. Practice for 5–20 rounds, depending on your comfort level.

VARIATIONS:

Torso rotation—Begin on all fours as you would in a Cat/Cow position. Inhale as you would normally in Cat Pose, then shift the torso towards the right side. Exhale, drop the belly down as you would in a Cow Pose, and then shift the torso over to the left side. Here you are making a counter-clockwise circle with the torso. Practice this torso rotation for 1 minute, and then repeat in a clockwise circle for another minute. This is a very animalistic variation, so let your body move fluidly like a fierce animal. You can also bend the elbows to help keep the motion flowing.

Tiger Pose—Begin in a neutral position on all fours with your knees under your hips and hands under your shoulders. Inhale and round your back like Cat Pose. Lift your right leg and bring your knee into your chest. Exhale and lift your head, slightly arch your back, and drop your belly like you would in Cow pose. Lift your right leg up and back, bending your knee, and pointing your toes up towards the sky. Repeat this motion slowly and steadily as you would in Cat/Cow for 10–30 *ujjayi* breaths.

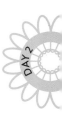

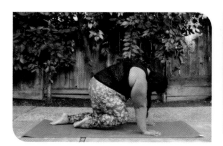 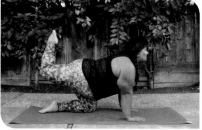

MOUNTAIN POSE AND PALM TREE POSE

(Tadasana)

ABOUT THE POSE:

The mountain is confident, strong, grounding, sturdy, and unwavering. Even though the pose may look simple, there is still action in Mountain Pose. It utilizes all of the elements of earth, fire, water, air, and ether. As well, the palm tree can grow to towering heights and still stand unwavering in a storm.

BODY BENEFITS:

Many of us are used to sitting hunched over on a daily basis, often unaware that we are even doing it. This pose can be used to improve our posture by lengthening the spine, and creating a grounded foundation by strengthening the thighs, knees, and ankles.

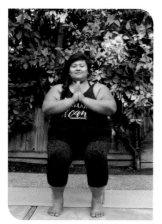

PROPS:

Even though these poses are practiced standing up, you can choose to take a seat in a chair if standing for a long period of time is difficult. Seat the sit bones at the edge of the chair so as to not use the backrest. Bend your knees and plant your feet on the ground. Sit as upright and tall as you can.

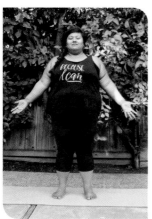

GET IN POSITION:

Come up to the front of your mat, with your feet hip-width apart. Your hands can be in a number of positions: palms together in prayer placed in front of the heart, placed down by the sides with palms facing forward, or arms raised above with palms together.

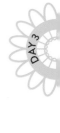

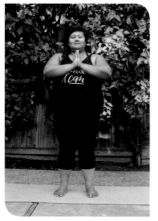

WHEN YOU ARE READY:

Root the soles of the feet firmly down into the ground. Stretch upward from the base of the tailbone all the way up to the crown of the head, lengthening and extending the spine. Activate all of the elements of the mountain—ground the feet, activate the fire of the legs, feel the fluidity of the spine, and reach up to the sky with your crown. Gaze ahead at your *drishti*, or shut the eyes, looking internally.

TRANSITION TO PALM TREE POSE:

With the feet hip-distance apart, reach your arms up overhead, interlacing your fingers together, and turning the palms to face the sky. Place the backs of your hands on top of the crown of your head. Inhale and lift the heels of your feet up off the floor, coming onto the balls of your feet; raise your interlaced palms up, reaching to the sky and elongating your body. Exhale, bringing your heels back down to the floor, and the tops of your hands down to the crown.

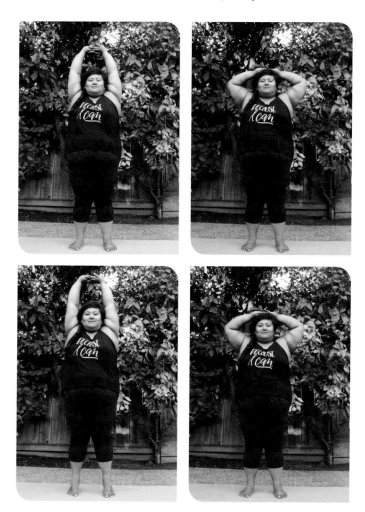

HOW LONG:

Mountain Pose: You can hold this pose for 20–30 deep *ujjayi* breaths, deepening your breath as you stand strong and tall.

Palm Tree Pose: Repeat the inhale and exhale motion, lifting up and down for 5–15 rounds. If coming onto the balls of your feet is difficult, repeat the motion with your arms only, keeping your feet flat and grounded.

VARIATION:

If you're feeling confident with Palm Tree Pose, why not try Swaying Palm Tree (*Tirya Tadasana*)? Keep the feet flat and grounded, hip-width apart, remaining strong and steady from the hips down. Inhale and raise your interlaced palms up. As you exhale, reach the palms over to your right side. Feel the length and stretch of the left side of your body. Inhale and bring the arms straight overhead; exhale, reaching over to the left side opening up the right side body. Repeat for 1 minute to the right and left at your own pace, feeling each side with the arms extended.

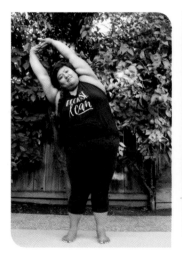
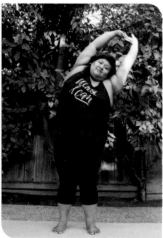

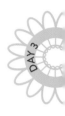

STANDING BACKBEND

(Anuvittasana)

ABOUT THE POSE:

We'd all love to be able to jump right into deep backbends like Wheel Pose (which we'll learn later), but having flexibility in your back usually comes later after long periods of practice. Before we can go further into a back-bending practice, we can start with a standing backbend. This is an accessible pose for anyone to practice.

BODY BENEFITS:

As the backbend deepens the front of the body opens up. Of course, backbends are great for the back, but this pose is also a big heart opener. Opening your heart has physical, mental, and spiritual benefits. This pose is great for opening yourself up and feeling more confident and less fearful. It's a great way to silence negative thoughts about yourself or your body. In addition to these great mental benefits, this pose strengthens the respiratory, cardiovascular, and endocrine (hormonal) systems.

PROPS:

This pose is mostly reliant on your own internal strength, but you can use a wall for support or balance. If standing is difficult for you, sit at the edge of a chair and don't use the backrest. Plant your feet on the floor hip-distance apart, or slightly wider for balance.

GET IN POSITION:

Stand at the front of the mat, feet hip-distance apart, and arms down by your side. Inhaling, reach the arms up straight overhead, fingertips reaching up towards the sky. Exhaling, take the gaze up between the hands. If you are not used to backbends and are still working on the uplift and lengthening of the spine, a good way to support the back from crunching is to place the hands, palms with fingers pointing down, on the lower back. Squeeze the shoulder blades together to open the heart. If you feel comfortable without the hands, they can also be placed palms together at your heart center.

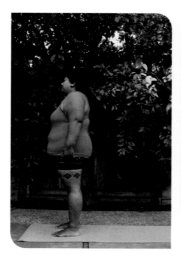
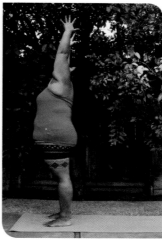

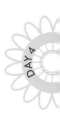

WHEN YOU ARE READY:

Ground your feet; lengthen your body from your kneecaps all the way to the tips of your fingers. Inhale and reach back with your arms, bringing the head back while moving your gaze behind you. Push the pelvis forward and squeeze the thighs and butt lightly as you arch the torso backward. Remember to engage the thighs and butt and lengthen the spine. Support the weight of the body in the arms as the back arches so you don't crunch the lower back. Only bend as far as feels natural. Don't force your back to go deeper than it can at the moment. It all takes time.

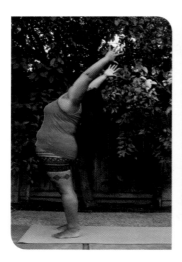
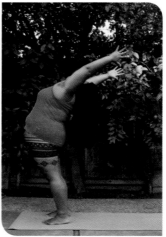

HOW LONG:

In backbends it is harder to expand the lungs and breathe deep into the chest, so when you are inhaling and exhaling breathe consciously into the lower part of the lungs. Hold the pose for 5-10 *ujjayi* breaths. You can also take your time repeating the pose in increments. You will probably find you can deepen your backbend by gradually extending the length of your hold. You can start off holding for 3 breaths, coming out of the pose, again for 5 breaths, exiting the pose, holding for 10 breaths, and exiting the pose. Hold it for as long as you feel comfortable without hurting yourself.

FORWARD FOLD

(Uttanasana)

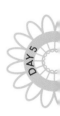

ABOUT THE POSE:

This is a pose to just relax and sink into, letting yourself enjoy the sensations. Even though this is a pose where there can be a deep and intense stretch in the hamstrings and calves, let your body melt and feel comfortably relaxed.

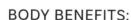

BODY BENEFITS:

This is a very therapeutic and revitalizing posture as it gives a boost of oxygen by allowing the blood to rush to the head instead of the feet as usual. It is a simple pose that can relieve stress, anxiety, depression, and fatigue. As you fold forward the spinal column lengthens, stretching the back muscles and stimulating the digestive and urogenital systems. It also strengthens the thighs and knees by stretching the hips, hamstrings, and calves.

PROPS:

It can take a while to fully reach the floor when practicing Forward Fold, so until then, using blocks is a good way to bring the floor up so you can have support. Place the blocks on the floor in front of your feet or wider. By placing your hands on the blocks, you create more points of connection with the floor so you feel stabilized. If you need more height, you can also use the edge of a chair.

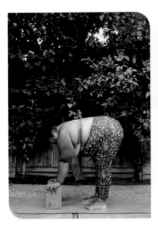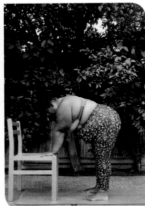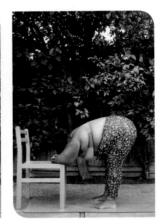

GET IN POSITION:

Stand at the front of your mat with feet hip-distance apart (blocks or chair placed in position for use). Inhale and sweep the arms up overhead.

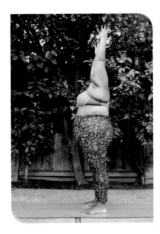

WHEN YOU ARE READY:

Exhale and slightly bend your knees. Bend forward at the hips and sweep the arms forward to drop the fingertips down to the floor or props, folding the upper body over the thighs and gazing down at the floor. You can keep the knees bent or extend them straight to activate the back leg muscles. To come out of the pose, inhale and bend your knees, sweeping your arms up and overhead. Then exhale, bringing your arms down by the sides.

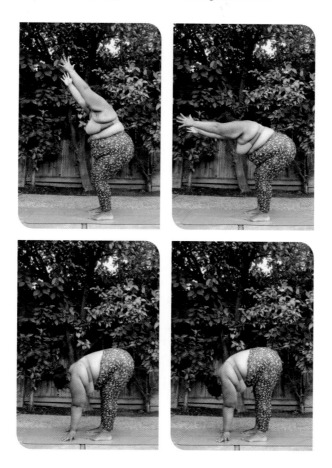

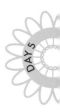

HOW LONG:

Hold the pose for 10–20 *ujjayi* breaths. Take your time feeling all the aspects of the pose.

VARIATIONS:

Bigger belly—If you have a belly that gets in the way, you can hold on to it, tuck it in towards the pelvis, or lift it up to make more space as you fold forward. You can also take the feet a little wider than hips distance apart to allow the belly to drop between the legs so you can feel the pose better.

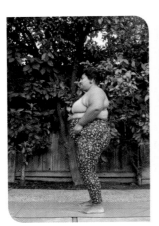 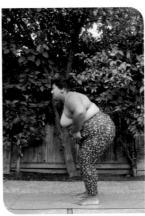 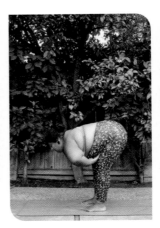 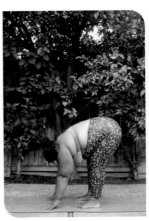

Ragdoll—Instead of dropping the hands to the floor, you can let gravity naturally lengthen the spine by grabbing on to each opposite elbow to ragdoll, swinging from side to side.

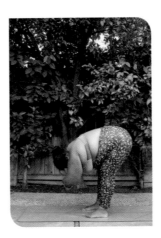

Arms behind back—Before you fold forward, interlace your fingers behind you (or hold on to a strap), tucking in the shoulder blades, opening the chest, and bending at the hips to fold forward, lifting the arms away from the back.

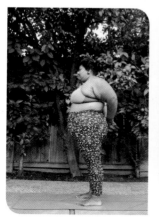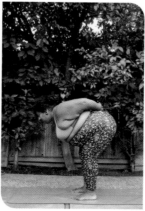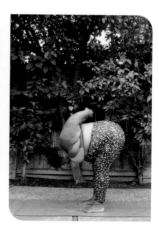

Swinging Forward Fold—To create more dynamic energy in this pose, raise the arms above the head, bend the knees, and in a fast motion sweep the arms down towards the floor, then reach them back behind while slightly straightening your legs. Bend the knees again and sweep the arms in a quick motion back up overhead while straightening the legs. Repeat this motion 5 or more times to feel more energetic. (See Kriya on page 19.)

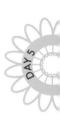

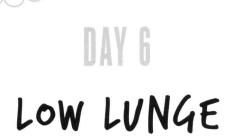

DAY 6

LOW LUNGE

(Anjaneyasana)

ABOUT THE POSE:

Low Lunge opens, strengthens, and stretches the body. It opens up the hips and frees blocked energy or emotion that we hold within us. Through Anjaneyasana, we are allowed to let go of the energies that don't serve us anymore and focus on the positive.

BODY BENEFITS:

When we spend a lot of time sitting, like at the office, it shortens our hip flexors and tightens the hip rotators, which can create pain in the hips and lower back. Practicing the lunge helps to counteract this by opening the hip to relieve tension, as well as strengthening the knees and stretching the hamstrings, quadriceps, and groin. This posture can even help relieve the pain of sciatica.

PROPS:

When first practicing this pose it can be hard to place your hands down on the floor while staying upright in the position. Using blocks can help keep your back in an upright position to avoid rounding of the spine. Place the blocks down on each side of your feet. Depending on your position they can move around to suit your needs. If you need a little more height, you can use two similar chairs, one on each side of you. Sometimes balance can throw you off as well—face a wall and place the big toe of your forward foot so it is touching the wall. This can help keep you steady. When doing a Low Lunge, the knee is directly on the floor and can sometimes hurt if the floor is not soft. You can place a folded blanket down underneath the knee for added comfort.

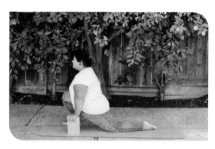
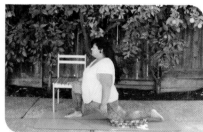

GET IN POSITION:

From a standing Forward Fold (Day 5), bend the knees to place the hands down onto the ground or blocks outside of the feet. Take the right leg back, in one big step or a couple small steps, and drop the knee down to the floor with the top of the right foot placed onto the mat. Keep the left knee pointing ahead of you with the shin perpendicular to the floor. If the left leg wants to open up to the left and not stay straight ahead, try using blocks to prop you up to stay aligned.

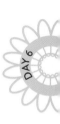

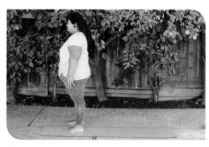
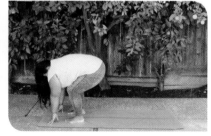

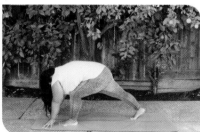
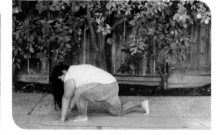

WHEN YOU ARE READY:

Slide the right leg back to open up the groin area. Inhale and lift the torso into an upright position with the chest open. Pull up with the crown of your head. Let your arms and hands drop by your sides and place them on the floor or blocks, or leave them hovering. Drop your pelvis down towards the mat, feeling the stretch in your hips and thighs.

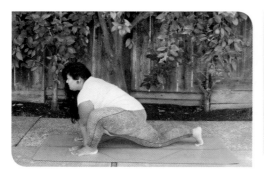
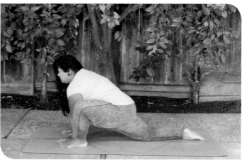
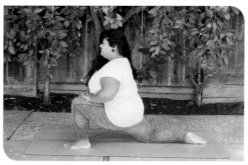

HOW LONG:

Hold the pose for 5–10 *ujjayi* breaths. It will take a while to bring the pelvis closer to the floor, so take your time slowly opening up the hips in increments. Start with holding the pose for 3 breaths, then 5 breaths, and then 10 breaths. Let yourself sink into the pose each time going as far as feels comfortable for you without pushing your muscles too fast.

VARIATIONS:

Crescent Lunge—This pose is a mix of the lunge and a standing backbend, with your bottom half lunging and your top half bending back. From the Low Lunge position, inhale and sweep the arms up and overhead. Reach the fingers up towards the sky and exhale, holding for a few moments. Inhale; reach up and backward, arching your back, pressing the pelvis forward and down towards the mat. The shape of your body, from your fingertips to the toes of your back foot, makes a crescent shape.

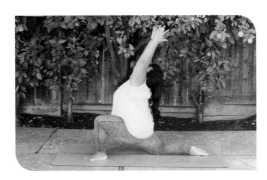

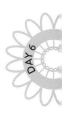

High Lunge—If being on the floor is difficult for you, you can opt to come into a High Lunge. Instead of dropping the knee down to the floor, stay up on the ball of the back foot. Still drop the pelvis down towards the floor, keeping the front knee pointing forward and the shin straight and perpendicular to the floor. Arms and hands can be dropped down by your side, or placed onto your hips. For extra support use two chairs, one on either side of your mat, placing a hand on each chair seat.

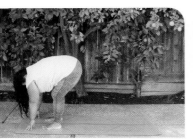
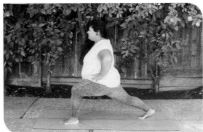
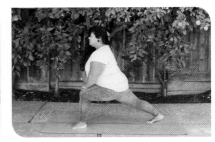

PLANK POSE AND FOUR-LIMBED STAFF POSE

(Uttihita Chaturanga Dandasana and Chaturanga Dandasana)

ABOUT THE POSE:

There is a lot of strength involved in practicing these poses. Through the strength you build here you will eventually be able to advance to more taxing arm balancing postures. That may seem far into the future of your practice now, but it is good to know that you are capable of getting there one day as you prepare your body for the new poses ahead.

BODY BENEFITS:

Both of these poses work on strengthening the wrists, arms, shoulders, and leg muscles. They also focus on the core muscles to help with stamina, and the back muscles along the spine to improve posture.

PROPS:

Balancing on the hands can put a lot of pressure on the wrists, so try placing a folded blanket just under the wrists to slightly angle the hands and relieve some pressure.

You can also place blocks underneath your hands to elevate your plank a bit higher, or use a chair if you would like more height in this pose. Pressure on the hands is still the same, but props can give you another way to practice higher off of the floor. If using the chair, place your hands onto the seat of the chair, walk the feet back, straightening the body until you are on the balls of the feet.

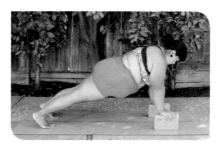

Even though traditionally the Plank and Four-Limbed Staff Pose are practiced on the floor, for some it can be difficult to get up and down. This pose can definitely be practiced using a wall in place of the floor while still feeling the benefits. Your arms should be shoulder-width apart, hands straight out in front against the wall with your fingers spread wide. Walk the feet back, coming onto the balls of the feet, keeping the whole backside straight and aligned. Stand 2–4 feet away from the wall (adjust to see what feels comfortable but will still challenge you).

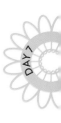

GET IN POSITION:

You can come into the pose from a Low/High Lunge by placing the hands down on the floor and stepping the front leg back to match the back leg. As well, you can begin the pose on all fours down on the mat with your hands placed directly under your shoulders, or using your preferred prop. Widen the fingers, extend the arms by pushing away from the floor, lengthen your neck muscles so that your head doesn't turtle into your shoulders, gaze down at the floor, and draw the abdominal muscles in to straighten the spine.

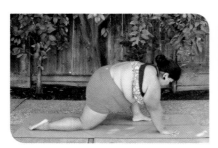
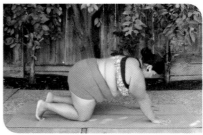

WHEN YOU ARE READY:

Tuck the toes, walking the feet back so that your body is a straight line from heel to head. You can also take a knee plank position by walking the legs back, and dropping the knees to the mat, making a straight line from the knees to the head. Press into the floor with your hands and engage the abdominal muscles to hold the body up off the ground.

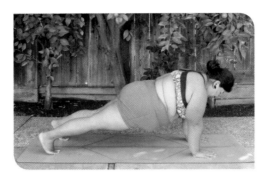

HOW LONG:

Since this is a great strengthening pose, you can practice holding for however long feels beneficial to you. Start off holding for 5–10 *ujjayi* breaths; then move on in increments to holding for 20 seconds, to 30 seconds, 1 minute, 2 minutes, till possibly 5 minutes. Breathe slowly and steadily, always staying aware of your breath.

TRANSITION TO FOUR-LIMBED STAFF POSE:

To move into Four-Limbed Staff Pose, or *Chaturanga Dandasana*, slowly lower the chest down towards the floor while keeping the arms tucked into the sides of the torso. Slowly come down to the mat, and try to avoid dropping the chest in a quick motion down to the floor. It's okay if your belly is touching the floor as you lower down, just keep your arms controlled until the front of the body is all the way down. Since this is a very challenging pose, another way of approaching it from Plank Pose is to drop the knees/chest/chin down to the floor one at a time. Then shimmy to drop the rest of the body down to the mat. This is more of a transitional pose so you don't have to hold it very long.

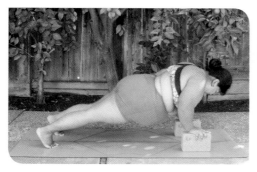
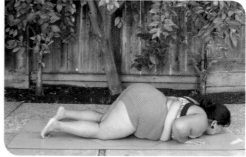

VARIATION:

Forearm Plank—This can be done on the floor or wall. Instead of balancing on the hands, which puts more pressure on the wrists, drop down to the forearms with the elbows directly underneath the shoulders. Press away from the floor with the forearms, engage the core, and lengthen the body into a straight line from the head to the heels.

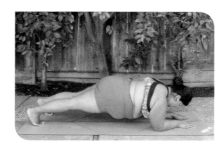

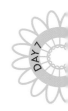

You can also do this pose on your knees, either from the start or by dropping to your knees from the full plank position. You should still maintain a straight line from your head down to your knees.

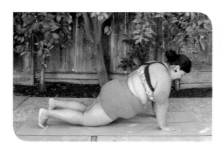
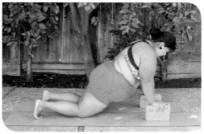

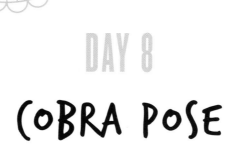

DAY 8

COBRA POSE

(Bhujangasana)

ABOUT THE POSE:

This pose represents the cobra rearing its hooded head. In traditional yoga texts the cobra is a symbol of immortality as it sheds its skin and is rejuvenated with new life. While practicing this pose focus on letting go of the past and moving forward with positivity.

BODY BENEFITS:

As you come into Cobra Pose, all of the muscles in the shoulders, chest, and abdomen are stretched and strengthened. This pose will decrease stiffness in the lower back, soothe symptoms of sciatica, and firm the butt. Cobra Pose is great for relieving stress and fatigue and improving blood circulation and digestion. It invigorates the heart, opens the lungs, and stimulates the kidneys, all while increasing flexibility in the spine.

PROPS:

If lying down on the floor is a bit difficult for you, you can practice Cobra Pose using a chair. There are two different ways to do this.

One way is to place the chair against the wall (this will stop it moving). Stand in front of the chair, dropping your hands down to the seat. The hand position can be either palms down with fingertips pointing forward, or hands gripping the sides of the seat; see which way feels comfortable for you. Walk the feet back staying on the balls of the feet, similar to approaching Plank Pose with a chair. Then drop the hips and arch the back as you would if you were down on the ground.

The second way of using the chair is to take a seat at the edge so you're not using the backrest. Ground the feet down into the floor a little wider than hip-width apart, and place your hands on your knees. Lift up with the crown of the head as the chest comes forward, feeling the arch in your spine. Ground the sit bones down into the chair as the chest presents forward. This way you can feel the benefit of the backbend even in a seated position.

Using the chair will have its benefits and disadvantages. Since you are not on the floor it won't stimulate the abdominal and pelvic muscles from the floor.

GET IN POSITION:

Lie face down on your mat. Place your hands palms down beneath your shoulders with your elbows bent and tucked into the sides of your torso. Spread your fingers wide.

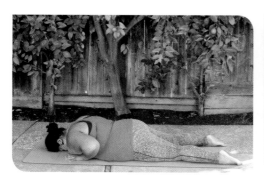
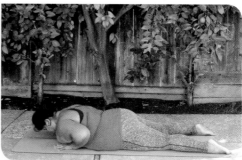

WHEN YOU ARE READY:

Press into the floor with the palms, pelvis, and tops of the feet, as you extend your arms. Inhale and lift the chest up off the floor to a height that feels comfortable to you; it could be 2 inches, 8 inches, or fully upright. Create a sense of lift with the crown of your head, lengthening your neck away from your shoulders, and feeling your spine lengthen all the way down to your tailbone. Press your pelvis into the floor and feel your buttocks firm. There should be no discomfort in your neck or lower spine as long as your vertebrae are straight and lengthened.

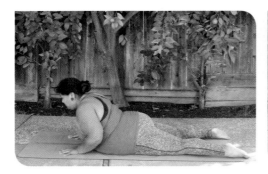 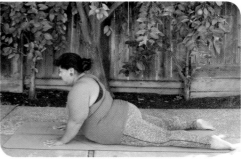

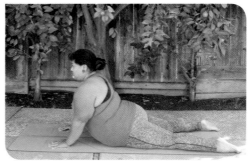

HOW LONG:

Inhale and exhale from the lower part of your lungs, keeping the breath slow and steady. Hold the pose for 10–20 *ujjayi* breaths. Then release back down to the mat.

VARIATIONS:

Sphinx Pose—If being down on the floor is okay for you but staying on the wrists for a long while is a bit difficult, drop your arms down to rest on your forearms and come into Sphinx Pose. Align your elbows underneath your shoulders, keeping your forearms straight out in front, with your palms down and fingers spread wide. Repeat as you would in Cobra Pose.

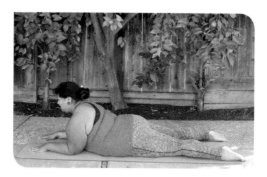

Cobra/Sphinx Twists—Whichever one of these poses you take, once you've come up into the pose, inhale, and as you exhale turn your head to the right and gaze back over towards your right foot. Hold the breath for 5 seconds. Inhale, and twist to face forward again, and then exhale, turning your head to the left and gazing over to your left foot. Hold the breath for 5 seconds, and inhale as you turn back and gaze ahead. You should feel an extra-nice twist as your head turns.

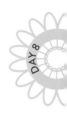

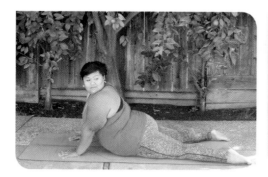 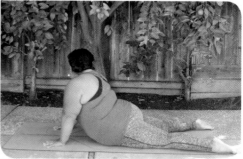

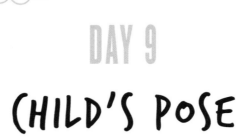

DAY 9

CHILD'S POSE

(Balasana)

ABOUT THE POSE:

Child's Pose is a reviving transitional pose. If during a yoga class (or life) you feel overwhelmed and find yourself breathing irregularly, take a moment to drop into Child's Pose. It can help calm the mind, slow the breath with awareness, and restore a sense of peace like that of a young child.

BODY BENEFITS:

Even though this seems like a passive pose, the body is still engaged. The hips, thighs, and ankles are stretched to help reduce stress and fatigue. The muscles across the front of your body relax as the back muscles passively stretch. This pose is also great for relieving back or neck pain.

PROPS:

This pose is practiced with the knees, shins, and tops of the feet resting on the floor as you sit back on the heels. If you need more cushioning to protect your legs, place a blanket over your mat. If sitting back on your heels is a bit difficult, roll up a blanket into a tube shape and place it behind your heels to sit back on. This pose asks you to place your forehead down on the floor, but sometimes it can be a bit difficult to reach the floor. Try placing a block or two in front to rest your forehead on. If you have a bolster or a firm pillow you can also place it lengthwise in front of you, to rest your upper body on.

If being on the floor completely is difficult for you, use a chair. Stand in front of the chair with your feet a little wider than hip-width apart. Inhale and raise your arms up and over. Exhale, bending your knees and dropping your hands down to the seat. Drop your chest down towards the floor, keeping the knees bent. Let yourself surrender in the pose.

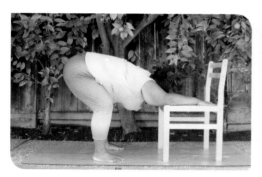 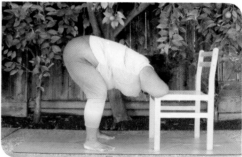

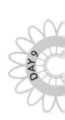

GET IN POSITION:

Come down onto your mat on all fours, tops of your feet on the mat, and bring your big toes together. Your knees can be together, or wider, about the width of your mat, to help accommodate a bigger belly. Then sit back on your heels. The hand position can vary depending on what feels comfortable for you when you come into the pose.

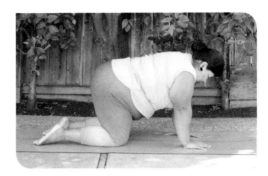

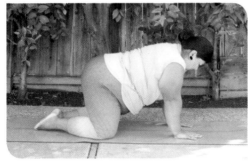

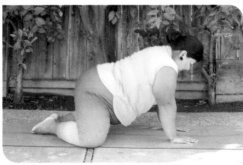

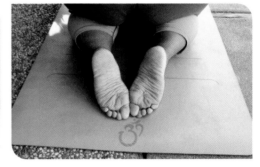

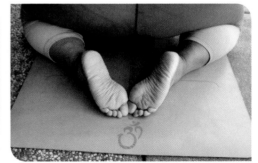

WHEN YOU ARE READY:

Walk the hands forward as you drop your belly down over the thighs or between your thighs, and drop the forehead and chest down towards your mat or prop. Your arms can be straight out in front with forearms and palms down on the mat, or you can stack your hands on top of each other and place them under your forehead, or leave them down by your sides. If your butt lifts up from your heels as you fold forward, it is completely fine. Just feel relaxed and take your time relaxing in the pose.

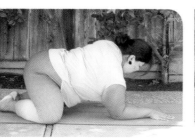
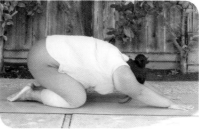
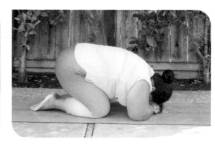
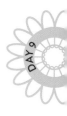

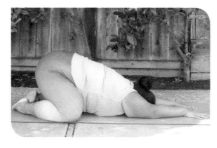
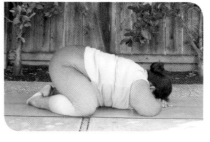

HOW LONG:

Hold the pose for 10–20 *ujjayi* breaths. In other yoga poses we normally breathe into the front of the body so the chest expands. But in this position we breathe and expand the back body using our back breathing (see page 65), so the lungs round the back.

DOWNWARD-FACING DOG

(Adho Mukha Svanasana)

ABOUT THE POSE:

This pose mimics the way dogs and other animals stretch their whole bodies. It is an essential pose in the Sun Salutations, and the most recognizable pose in yoga. Downward Dog can be a resting pose or a transitional pose and is a mild inversion strength builder because it allows you to have the sensation of being upside down as you build the upper body strength.

BODY BENEFITS:

Practicing Downward Dog every day can help energize the body by increasing blood flow to the brain to calm the nervous system. Physically it stretches the hands, shoulders, spine, hamstrings, calves, and arches of the feet, as well as building strength in the arms, shoulders, and legs. This pose can even relieve headaches, back pain, and fatigue, while relieving the brain of stress and depression.

PROPS:

To relieve pressure from the wrists in this pose, place a folded blanket directly beneath the wrists to elevate them and shift the pressure onto the fingers. You can also place a set of blocks underneath your hands to give a little more elevation in the pose. If being on the floor is difficult, place a chair facing away from you, place your hands on the top of the backrest, walk your feet back, and drop your head down between your arms, bringing the chest down towards the floor. Come into an inverted L shape, back flat and parallel to the floor and the legs slightly bent or straight. This can also be done with the edge of a table. If there are no props around, stand about 2-3 feet away from a wall, place your hands on the wall, and walk your hands down to come into an L shape.

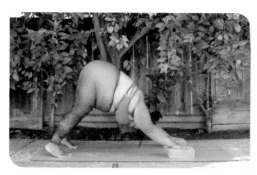
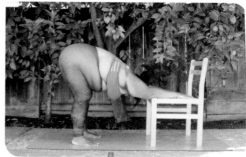

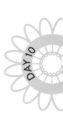

GET IN POSITION:

Begin on all fours, with or without props, placing the hands down with fingers wide, and tucking your toes underneath. Press your palms, fingers, and balls of your feet firmly into the mat. Inhale and lift your knees an inch or two up off the ground, and hold for a few moments to feel the sensations on the hands and feet.

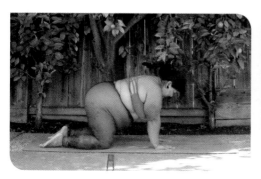
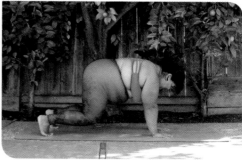

WHEN YOU ARE READY:

Exhale; as you lift the butt up towards the sky, drop the chest down towards the mat, and pull your hips up and back, straightening the arms and legs. Drop your heels towards the floor. Press away from the floor with equal pressure in your hands and feet to lift up with your hips, extending your spine and firming your thighs. Keep your arms straight without locking your elbows, and your head between your upper arms with your neck extended so your head does not hang or turtle into the shoulders.

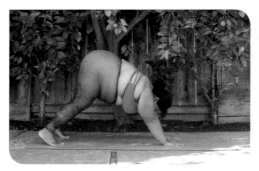 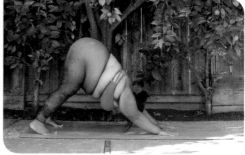

It's more important that the arms are straight and aligned with the back and spine than it is to have the legs fully extended and straight. So bend the knees as much as you need until your flexibility increases and you can fully extend them.

HOW LONG:

Hold for 10–20 *ujjayi* breaths. If you need to take a moment to drop down to the knees and rest from the pose, do it! Take your time and come back into the pose to go a little deeper than you did before.

VARIATIONS:

Dolphin Pose—If you can be on the floor but your wrists are still bugging you drop your elbows down and rest on your forearms. Keep your arms shoulder-distance apart with your palms down and fingers spread wide.

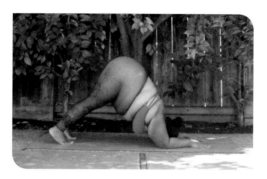

Puppy Pose—This pose is a mix of Child's Pose and Downward Dog and could be a step between the poses to prepare you for Downward Dog. Begin on all fours, knees underneath and hip-distance apart. Slowly walk the hands forward and drop the chest down to the floor. Extend your arms out in front, chest touching the floor, back slightly arched, hips up with your butt in the air, and thighs perpendicular to the floor.

Three-Legged Downward-Facing Dog—Once you feel comfortable practicing this pose, you can alternate lifting each foot off the ground. Keep your hips squared and aligned. Lift your foot, creating a long line all the way from the sole of your foot, down your back, through the crown of your head, and down to your hands.

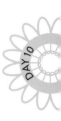

DAY 10

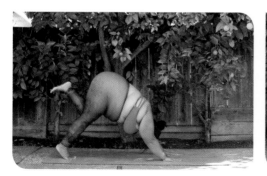

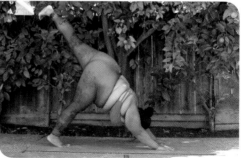

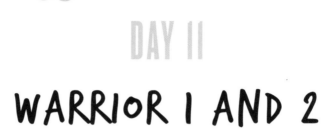

DAY 11

WARRIOR 1 AND 2

(Virabhadrasana)

ABOUT THE POSE:

The warrior poses were named after the warrior Virabhadra, the incarnation of the Hindu god Shiva. The poses embody the fierce and powerful strength of the warrior—balancing power, strength, focus, and stability in all aspects of life. Practicing the warrior series can help you find the strength to overcome obstacles of the physical, mental, emotional, and spiritual varieties.

BODY BENEFITS:

These are strong standing poses that engages the whole body to develop stamina, balance, and concentration. The whole front side of your body—neck, chest, belly, groin—is being stretched. Your lungs expand to improve the breath and bring more oxygen to the body. These poses also strengthens the shoulders, arms, back muscles, thighs, calves, and ankles.

PROPS:

These are balancing poses, so if balance isn't a strong point for you just yet, try standing next to a wall and placing a hand against it to keep you steady. You can also try facing a wall with your front foot toes just touching the surface. Touching the wall with the front foot toes helps to stabilize your balance. If you don't have a clear wall to use, place two chairs by your sides facing away from you. Holding on to the top of the backrests will give you some security when balancing in the pose.

GET IN POSITION:

If you are practicing your flow of Days 1–13, from Downward-Facing Dog, lift the right leg up into a Three-Legged Downward-Facing Dog, and sweep the right foot forward, bringing the right foot to the floor between the hands. This sweep can be in multiple steps walking the foot forward until the foot is between the hands. From here, lift the hands up from the floor, arms by your sides, bringing the torso into an upright position.

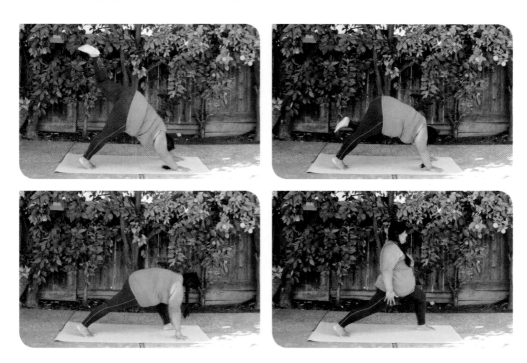

If you want to come into the pose without the transition, begin standing at the front of your mat. Take a big step back with your right foot so your legs are in an upside down V shape about 2–4 feet apart. Keep your hips squared facing forward, each foot in line with its respective hip, and toes pointing forward. Inhale, gazing ahead. Raise your arms up and over your head with your fingertips reaching to the sky, or placed on the hips.

WHEN YOU ARE READY:

Exhale and drop your hips straight down, keeping your hips and shoulders aligned with each other. Bend your front knee to align over your ankle, keep your shin perpendicular to the floor and your back leg straight with the back foot heel up off the floor or sole of the foot flat on the floor. Your back leg or foot may need to turn outward for comfort, and that's okay. Press your feet down into the mat as the arches of the feet lift. Sink your pelvis down, opening the hips. Push your chest forward and lift up with the crown of your head, and lengthen the body as the arms reach straight up. Stand strong like the warrior.

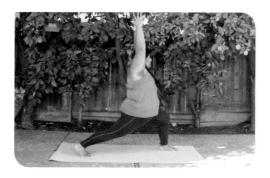

TRANSITIONING TO WARRIOR 2:

From Warrior 1 inhale and lift your hips back up, straightening the legs into an inverted V and pivot the back foot so that your toes are pointing outward. Rotate your torso to the right as well, facing outward. Drop your hips down, bending the original front knee again, keeping your front knee over your ankle. Sweep your right arm back over the back leg, and bring your left arm forward over the front leg. The arms are aligned with one another in one straight line parallel to the floor. Gaze ahead over the left arm, open the chest, and sink your pelvis down opening your hips. Feel powerful in Warrior 2. Exit the pose by lifting your hips up into the inverted V and stepping your back foot forward next to your front foot. Repeat Warrior 1 and 2 on the opposite side.

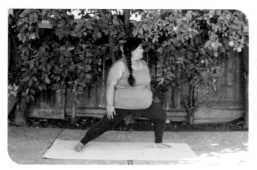 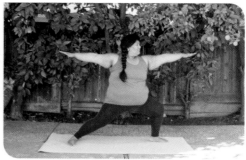

HOW LONG:

Hold Warrior 1 for 10–20 *ujjayi* breaths, transition into Warrior 2, and hold for another 10–20 *ujjayi* breaths.

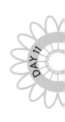

WIDE-LEGGED FORWARD FOLD

(Prasarita Padottanasana)

ABOUT THE POSE:

This straddled pose is a soothing one to practice after a more vigorous standing yoga practice, cardio, running, or cycling. Fully relaxing in the pose can release tension, stress, anxiety, mild depression, and stiffness. This pose is also helpful for preparing the body for inversions like handstand or headstand.

BODY BENEFITS:

In this pose the muscles in the back and inner legs are being stretched and strengthened. As the spine lengthens the hips open to relieve mild back pain and stimulate the internal abdominal organs. Depending on the arm position, this fold can also relieve neck and shoulder tension.

PROPS:

Dropping the hands down to the floor fully might take some time, so you can use either a chair or blocks to help prop yourself higher in the pose. Place the block(s) down in front of you, holding on to them for height and support. When using a chair, drop down to your hands, or elbows and forearms, to fold deeper while remaining in a standing position.

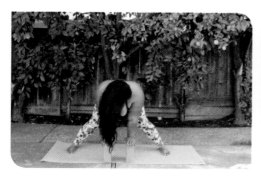 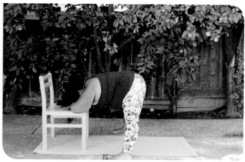

GET IN POSITION:

Begin in a standing position, facing the long side of your mat. Step the left foot 1–2 feet to the left and the right foot 1–2 feet to the right. Take a wide stance that feels comfortable for you, with your toes pointing ahead. Keep your knees slightly bent so that the knee joints do not lock straight. Place your hands on your hips, or inhale reaching the hands up overhead.

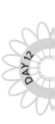

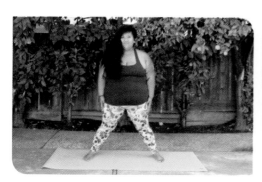 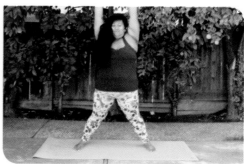

WHEN YOU ARE READY:

Inhale, and hold for a moment. Exhale, and bend forward at the hips. Drop your torso to bring your chest forward and the crown of your head down towards the floor. Fold as far as you can without discomfort. If you have a bigger belly, you can lift it up and away from you as you come into the pose to give you more room to fold forward. Drop your hands down to any arm variation you like: touching your fingertips to the floor or prop, holding on to opposite elbows, or touching the tops of the feet. Let your torso naturally hang down from your hips, keeping the legs upright and hips aligned with ankles. As you inhale lengthen the spine, and as you exhale fold deeper into the pose. To come out of the pose bend the knees more, and place your hands onto your hips. Use your legs to lift your torso back to an upright position. Step the feet back together into Mountain Pose.

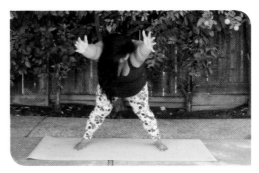

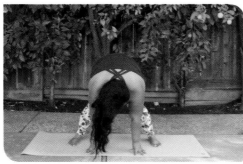
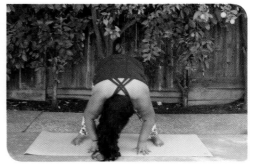

HOW LONG:

Hold for 30 seconds to 2 minutes, allowing yourself to let go and relax while staying active in the leg muscles.

VARIATION:

A great variation on this pose is the twist. With your arms dropped down to the floor or props, inhale and place your right hand down on the floor directly in front of your face. Exhale and raise your left arm up, twisting the torso towards the left side. Gaze up towards your left hand to help with the twist. Hold for 20–30 seconds, then bring the left arm back down, and repeat on the right side.

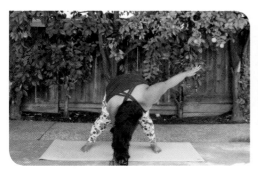
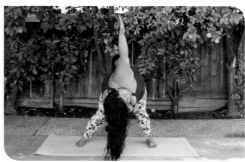

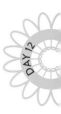

If you want to challenge yourself more in this pose while opening your chest and shoulders, try this arm variation with your hands clasped behind the back. Beginning in a standing wide-legged position, clasp and interlace your fingers behind your back (or hold on to a strap to get your hands as close together as possible). Bend your knees and bend at the hips to fold forward. Your shoulder blades should pull closer together as you lift your clasped hands up away from your back, feeling your chest and shoulders open up deeper. Hold for 10–30 seconds, then bend your knees and lift the torso into an upright position.

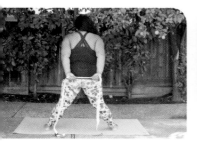
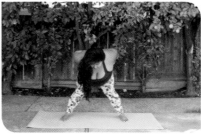
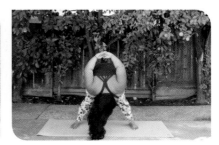

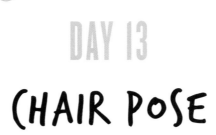

DAY 13

CHAIR POSE

(Utkatasana)

ABOUT THE POSE:

Also known as Awkward Chair Pose because you are attempting to sit down on nothing, this pose can be described as fierce and powerful because you will definitely feel your thighs burning and heart pumping!

BODY BENEFITS:

Chair Pose strengthens the feet, ankles, Achilles tendons, calves, shins, hip flexors, and back. It also stimulates the internal digestive system to help with metabolism and increases the heart rate.

PROPS:

Using the stability of the wall is a good way to practice. Stand in a neutral position, resting your hips and butt against the wall, with your back and arms away from the wall. Slowly walk your feet forward about 1-2 feet (going only as far as a thigh length away from the wall), and lower your hips down the wall, taking a seat. Plant your feet down, press the hips into the wall, and raise the arms up and forward.

GET IN POSITION:

Stand at the front of your mat in a neutral standing position with your feet hip-distance apart. Inhale and raise your arms up overhead, fingertips reaching to the sky, and neck and spine lengthening. Keep your gaze straight ahead at your *drishti*.

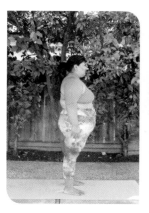
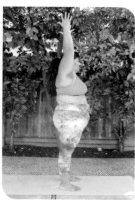

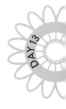

DAY 13

WHEN YOU ARE READY:

Exhale and bend your knees so they hover over your toes as you drop your tailbone towards the floor. Your thighs should be parallel to the floor, or as close to parallel as you can manage. Lean your chest forward for a slight arch in your back. Keep your arms extended forward at a 45-degree angle to your thighs, creating a straight line from your tailbone, up the spine, and all the way to the tips of your fingers.

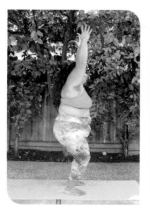
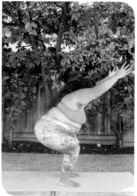

HOW LONG:

Hold for 10–30 *ujjayi* breaths. The longer you hold this pose the more stamina you build in your legs. Keep practicing so that you can hold the pose for longer each time. Keep your breath steady, slow, and controlled.

VARIATION:

You can change up the chair pose by adding a twist. From Chair Pose, inhale and bring your palms together in prayer hands in front of your heart. Exhale and from the tailbone up to the crown of the head, rotate the torso towards the right side, feeling a twist in the spine. Bring your left elbow to rest over your right thigh (if your elbow doesn't go that far that's okay; as long as you feel the twist in the spine you will feel the benefit of the pose). You can also drop the left hand to the floor, with the fingertips just grazing it, and reach the right arm up overhead. Inhale and come back to center. Exhale, twisting over to the left side. Hold each side for 10–30 breaths.

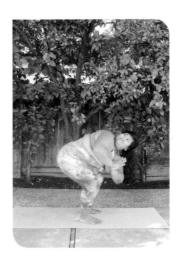

FLOW DAYS 1-13 POSES

HOW TO TRANSITION:

Among the different yoga practices, the speed at which we practice flows can vary. If you are just starting out, take your time transitioning from one pose to the next. This is not a race to see who can finish fastest. Especially in a home practice by yourself it is beneficial to take your time feeling each pose and getting the full benefits without having to rush through movements.

The thirteen poses that we practiced over the past two weeks are arranged here so that you can naturally transition from pose to pose.

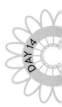

+ Warm-Ups > Cat Pose/Cow Pose

+ Cat Pose/Cow Pose > Mountain Pose

+ Mountain Pose > Palm Tree Pose

+ Palm Tree Pose > Standing Backbend

+ Standing Backbend > Forward Fold

+ Forward Fold > Low Lunge

+ Low Lunge > Plank Pose

+ Plank Pose > Four-Limbed Staff Pose

+ Four-Limbed Staff Pose > Cobra Pose

+ Cobra Pose > Child's Pose

+ Child's Pose > Downward-Facing Dog

+ Downward-Facing Dog > Warrior 1

+ Warrior 1 > Warrior 2

+ Warrior 2 > Wide-Legged Forward Fold

+ Wide-Legged Forward Fold >
  Chair Pose

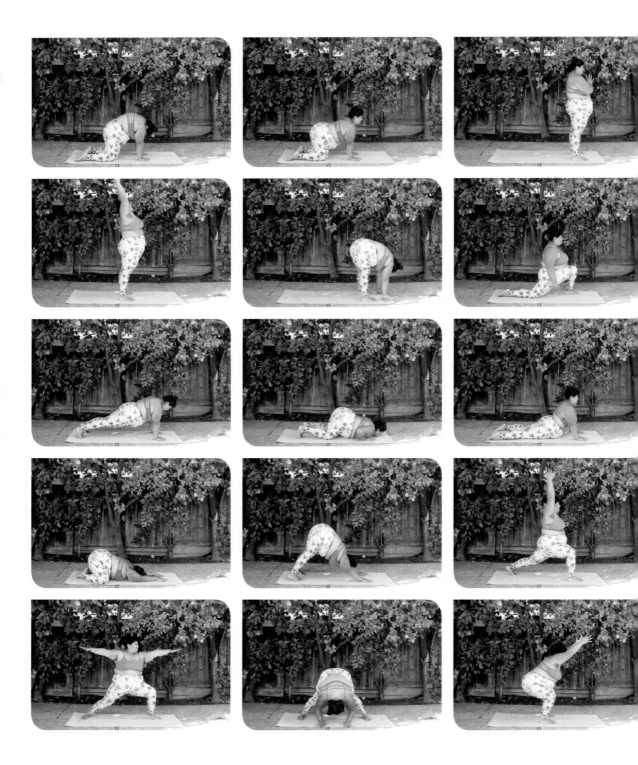

PROPS:

Whenever you are practicing a flow, it is good to have all your props ready to go next to your mat. Even if you don't end up using them, they are within arm's reach and there to help you out. If you know you need a wall, practice next to the wall. Have your chair out and ready, blocks set up on each side of you, one or two straps, blankets or bolsters. Have them all out ready to use when the time is right.

MAKE ADJUSTMENTS:

If something doesn't feel right, take the time to physically move things around. Sometimes my belly gets in the way when I want to go deeper into a pose, so I lift it up and move it to open up more space. If transitioning from a pose in one big step is difficult, break that big step into smaller steps. Be kind to yourself and your body; we are not all able to adapt to new things quickly. Our bodies have to take time to learn with repeated motions. You are also allowed to stop and drop into a Child's Pose (see Day 9) whenever the buildup of energy is a bit overwhelming. Take a moment to catch your breath and then keep going.

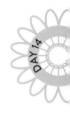

EXTENDED TRIANGLE POSE

(Utthita Trikonasana)

ABOUT THE POSE:

The triangle is one of the strongest shapes because its weight is balanced evenly throughout. In Triangle Pose we find the strength and stability to balance ourselves.

BODY BENEFITS:

Physical and mental balance and stability can be gained from practicing Triangle Pose. The hamstrings, groin, and hips are deeply stretched to help relieve back pain, stress, and sluggish feelings. It also brings strength to the thighs, hips, and back and is therapeutic for anxiety and sciatica.

PROPS:

It might take a while to be able to touch the floor in this pose. Place a block or two next to the inside of the ankle you will be leaning towards, so that when you drop your hand down you will have support. If you feel you need some more height, use a chair facing inward over the foot. If you are practicing without other props but want more support, try standing with your back to a wall, lightly touching it. The wall will be there if you feel like you might fall out of the pose, but gives you your space to find the strength and balance within yourself.

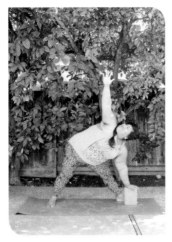
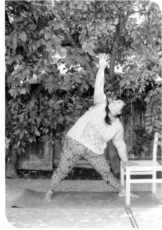

GET IN POSITION:

Begin in a wide-legged stance on the mat. Pivot your right foot so that the toes are pointing outward to the right, while keeping your heels aligned with one another (place your prop down if you need it). Inhale and raise your arms up and out to the sides, parallel to the floor, with palms facing down. Exhale and turn your head right to gaze over your right hand. At the hips, lean your torso sideways over your right thigh. Your right hand should reach as far right as you can manage while still keeping the arms straight and parallel to the floor.

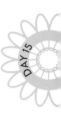

DAY 15

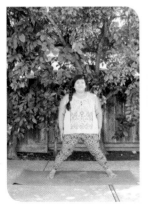
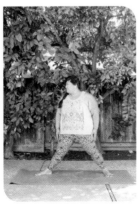
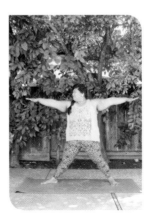
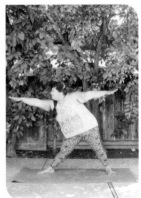

WHEN YOU ARE READY:

Keeping your arms straight and aligned with each other, drop your right hand down to the floor, prop, on the shin or foot, or hovering on the inside of the right foot as you bend sideways. Root the right hand down for stability, as the left arm reaches upward to the sky, so the hands are reaching away from each other. Gaze forward or up at your left hand. Keep your legs straight but not locked at the knees.

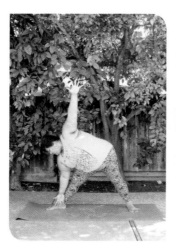 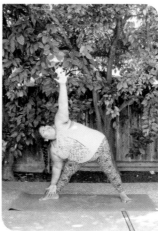

HOW LONG:

Hold for 10–30 *ujjayi* breaths. Then come back out of the pose the way you came into it. Lift the torso and arms back up parallel to the floor, at the hips shift the torso into an upright position, and pivot the right foot so it is pointing forward. Then repeat Triangle Pose again on the left side.

VARIATION:

Revolved Triangle Pose—From Triangle Pose on the right side, drop the left arm down to the floor or prop to meet the right hand. Plant the left hand down on the floor or prop to support the body, and raise the right arm up, reaching the fingers to the sky as the torso twists towards the right. Gaze back behind you as the spine lengthens and twists. Hold for 10–30 breaths, then repeat on the left side.

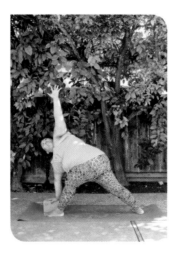

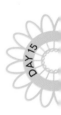

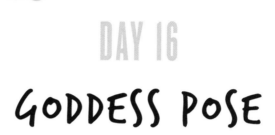

GODDESS POSE

(Utkata Konasana)

ABOUT THE POSE:

A goddess is more than just a mythical deity. She represents embracing the universal feminine energy within us, the Shakti. Whether you are a woman or a man, having both the feminine and masculine energies helps us to find balance in the soft and the hard. Goddess Pose is about finding that balance of energies, and this fierce squat brings the feminine energy by opening the hips.

BODY BENEFITS:

In this pose, the whole lower body is activated and strengthened, warming up the lower back, glutes, hips, thighs, calves, and ankles. At the same time the chest is opening, stimulating the respiratory system and lengthening the spine. This pose is great for improving balance, focus, and concentration.

PROPS:

For some support and guidance, you can straddle a chair. As you come down into the pose, the seat of the chair will be your guide. You can hover above it or sit down. If your knees are sensitive to bending, this is a good way to still feel the stretch in your hips without hurting your knees. This pose can be done with your heels lifted, balancing on the balls of your feet. If you find this a bit difficult, try placing a rolled-up blanket under your heels. A wall can also be a useful prop in this pose—stand with your back to the wall, 1–2 inches away, and use it for support for balance.

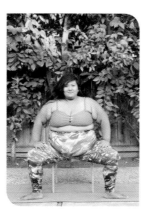

GET IN POSITION:

Begin in a wide-legged stance with your feet about 3 feet apart, lengthwise on your mat. Pivot both of your feet outward as far as feels comfortable, keeping your ankles aligned with each other. Inhale and raise your arms up overhead with your palms facing forward, or begin with your hands placed on top of your thighs.

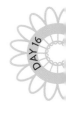

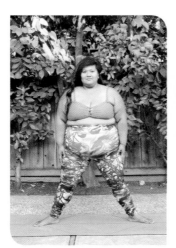
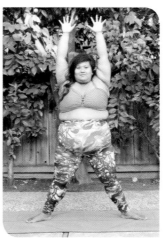

WHEN YOU ARE READY:

Exhale and bend your knees so they are aligned over your ankles. Drop your hips down into a hovered seat, with your thighs as parallel to the floor as you can manage so that it feels comfortable but challenging. Bend your arms at the elbows at a 90-degree angle so your upper arms are parallel to the floor. Spread your fingers wide, and press your shoulder blades together to open up your chest. Lengthen your spine, reaching up with the crown of your head. Plant your feet into the floor. For an extra challenge lift your heels up off the floor coming onto the balls of the feet.

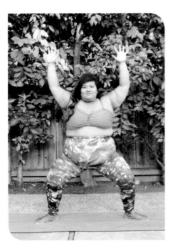 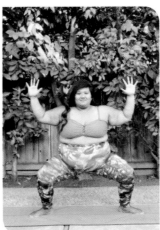 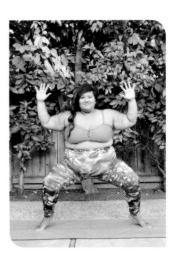

HOW LONG:

Hold for 10–30 *ujjayi* breaths like the fierce goddess you are.

VARIATIONS:

Twists—Begin in Goddess Pose with your hands on top of your thighs. Exhale. From your hips turn your torso to the left, bringing the right shoulder down and to the center in front of you. Gaze back over your left shoulder, increasing the twist. Hold for 10–20 breaths. Come back to the original pose. On your next exhale repeat on the right side.

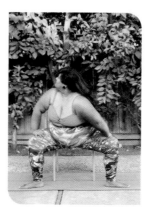

Spider Pose—Begin in Goddess Pose with your hands on top of your thighs. Exhale and bend at your hips, folding forward. Drop your chest down between your legs and cross your arms, making an X on the ground with the tops of the hands down on the floor. Hold for 10–20 breaths and lift back up out of the pose.

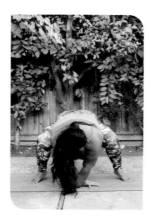

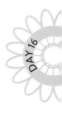
DAY 16

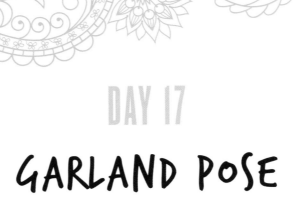

GARLAND POSE

(Malasana)

ABOUT THE POSE:

Garlands of flowers are made for ritual offerings, and prayer beads (*mala*) are used for spiritual and meditative practices. We use hip-opening poses to prepare the body for long periods of meditation. Sitting for long periods of time can shorten hip flexibility by creating tightness in the hip flexors, thighs, and groin. By practicing hip openers such as Garland Pose, we can allevi-ate hip and lower back problems that throw off our balance.

BODY BENEFITS:

As well as stretching the muscles of the torso, hips, groin, thighs, and ankles, Garland Pose can aid in digestion and elimination, as well as increasing the flow of blood to the pelvis.

PROPS:

If you are not used to squatting, the automatic reflex is for your heels to come up. It will take time to get both your heels and hips down at the same time, so be patient with yourself. If you would like more support so that you are not just balancing on the balls of the feet, place a rolled-up blanket under your heels so your foot has even pressure on both the ball and heel. In the pose, you will want to try to keep the heels down, so plant the soles of the feet down to the ground. For more support once you've dropped your butt down in the pose, place one or two blocks between your feet slightly back. You can rest your sit bones down on the block(s) so your weight is not all on your legs. Another option is to use a small step stool; while this isn't a traditional yoga prop, it has a lot more surface area on which to place your sit bones. Stacking props on top of each other is a good way to get more height as well.

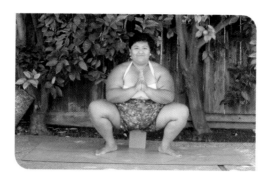

GET IN POSITION:

Stand at the front of your mat in a neutral position. Take a wide stance with your feet about the width of your mat apart, feet slightly turned outward. Place any props you might be using within reach or in place already. Inhale and bring the palms of your hands together in a prayer position in front of your heart.

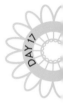

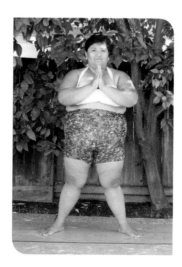

WHEN YOU ARE READY:

Exhale and bend your knees, dropping your hips down. Squat as low as you can go while keeping your heels on the floor as best you can. Be comfortable wherever you are in the position, just slightly squatting, all the way down on your prop, or in full *Malasana*. It will take time to come into a full Garland Pose, so be patient and kind to yourself. If you are all the way down, place your elbows just inside your knees and lift up with the crown of your head, lengthening your spine. To come out of the pose, you can come straight up from the squat, or place your hands down in front of you on the floor. Straighten your legs into a Forward Fold, keeping your knees slightly bent as you roll your spine upright vertebrae by vertebrae until you are fully upright.

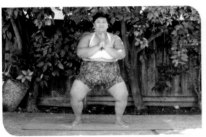 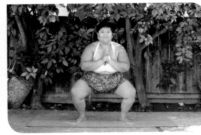 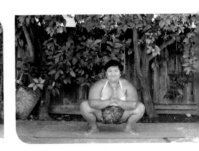

HOW LONG:

Hold for 10 seconds to 1 minute, keeping your breath calm and steady.

VARIATION:

Twists—Begin in Garland Pose. From prayer hands, drop your right hand down to the floor in front of the right foot, and raise your left arm, reaching up and back. Reach your left arm and shoulder back, squeezing your shoulder blades together to open up your chest, gazing up at the left hand. Hold for 10–30 breaths, then repeat on the right side.

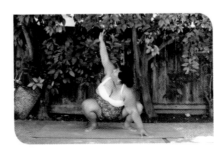

TREE POSE

(Vrksasana)

ABOUT THE POSE:

When standing tall in this pose, you are like the strong tree gently swaying in the wind and rooted down into the earth. While in this pose think about nature and the sprouting of new life.

BODY BENEFITS:

Tree Pose stretches and builds strength through the whole body—all the way from the bottom of the feet to the top of the head. It helps to focus, balance, and coordinate the body and mind. When you are able to focus, you are able to achieve a true meditative state.

PROPS:

It will take a while to find a steady balance in this pose. As you practice Tree Pose, stand next to a wall or place a chair by your side. Try not to rely too heavily on props for balance so that you can improve your own natural balancing skills. Hover your hand over the top of the chair or an inch or two away from the wall, placing your fingertips on the props when you feel off balance.

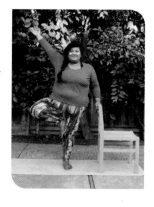

GET IN POSITION:

Stand at the front of your mat in a neutral standing position. Spread the toes of your right foot out, rooting all of the toes and sole of foot into the ground. Shift your weight over to your right foot, so that it is carrying most of your weight. Bend your left knee and lift your left foot up off the ground, bringing your thigh parallel to the floor in front of you. Take a moment to find your balance here, and feel the weight of your body balancing on one point.

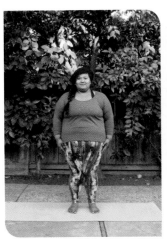 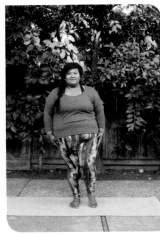 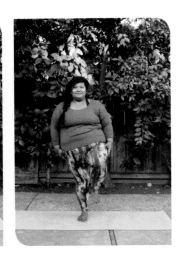

WHEN YOU ARE READY:

Swing your leg to the left, opening up your inner thigh. Place your left foot on the inside of your right leg: either on the ankle, calf, or inner thigh. Avoid placing your foot next to your knee joint because the joint is not stable. You can also grab hold of your ankle to place your foot where you want. Root your right foot down in the ground, finding a steady balance by activating the muscles of the calf and thigh. Lift up from your pelvis all the way to the crown of your head, expanding the branches of the mind out and up. As you find balance, feel the sway of your body like a tree moving in the wind. If you fall out of balance, just get right back in positon. If you find steadiness in Tree Pose, you can bring the hands together in prayer position or reach your arms up overhead, sprouting the arms and fingers like branches out to the sky. Exit the pose by lifting your foot away from your right leg, bringing your left knee ahead of you, and dropping the foot back down to the ground. Shake out your legs, and repeat on the opposite side.

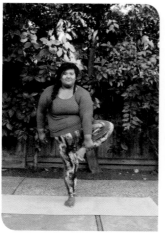
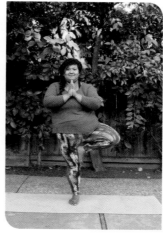

HOW LONG:

Once you find balance, hold the pose for 10–30 *ujjayi* breaths. Take the time to find comfort in your body and mind, and meditate in the pose.

VARIATION:

Begin in Tree Pose, balancing on your right foot. Raise your arms up and over, bringing your palms together again over your head. At the hips, lean over towards your left side, opening up the body's right side, and finding new balance in the Swaying Tree Pose. Hold for 10–30 breaths and come back out of the pose. Repeat on the opposite side.

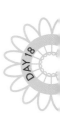

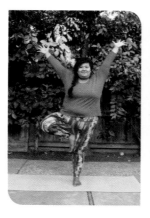
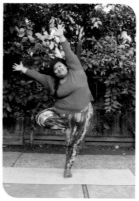

KING DANCER POSE

(Natarajasana)

ABOUT THE POSE:

Dancer Pose is a balancing and back-bending pose that brings strength, openness, and elegance inspired by the "Dance of Shiva." Shiva is one of the principal deities in Hinduism, and his dance represents the energies of creation and destruction. Balance in the movement to become still in the pose and find peace and calm.

BODY BENEFITS:

Through this pose you build strength, flexibility, coordination, and focus in the whole body. In Dancer Pose, the shoulders, chest, and hips are all being stretched and strengthened, while the back muscles are developing flexibility around the spine to help improve your posture.

PROPS:

Reaching your hand all the way to your foot can be difficult, but using a strap can help. There are different ways to attach the strap. One way is to loop one end around the ball of your foot or ankle, and tighten the buckle so that it doesn't slip. Another method is to hold each end of the strap looping the middle around the ball of your foot. The third option is to loop the middle of the strap around the back of your ankle, then bring the two ends together over the top of your foot, placing the strap in between the big toe and second toe. Bring the strap back under the foot to the heel, bend your knee bringing your foot towards your butt cheek, and swing the rest of the strap over your shoulder.

If the balance on the foot feels a little shaky, grab on to the back of a chair, or stand close to wall for support until it feels comfortable to let go.

GET IN POSITION:

Begin standing at the front of your mat. Shift the weight of your body over to your left foot, finding your center of balance. Slowly lift up your right foot, bending your knee out in front of you. Loop the strap or grab on to your ankle or foot, bringing your right heel to your right butt cheek. Establish your balance, and lift your left arm straight up overhead with your fingertips reaching to the sky. Your arm will be the counterbalance in this pose.

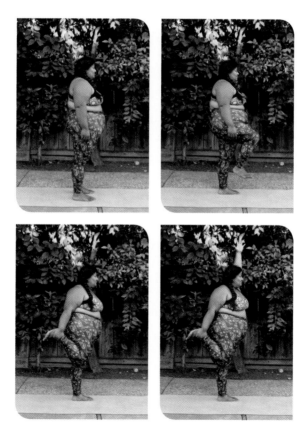

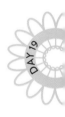

WHEN YOU ARE READY:

Kick your right foot back, lifting your leg to bring your right thigh parallel to the floor. At the same time, drop your torso forward, reaching your left hand out in front of you. Lift the chest and arms up. Create more space between the back leg, back, and arm. Try not to let your right knee splay out to the side, keeping the leg aligned with the hips. Focus on pressing down through your tailbone to avoid stressing your lower back.

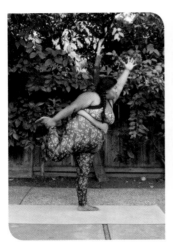 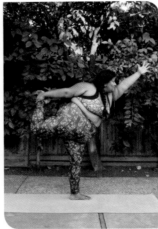 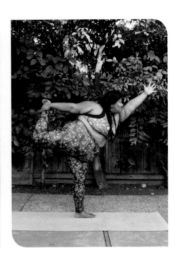

HOW LONG:

Hold for 10–30 *ujjayi* breaths, staying as steady as you can. If you fall out of the pose, come back into it, continuing your breaths. Exit the pose and repeat on the opposite side.

DAY 20

HALF MOON POSE

(Ardha Chandrasana)

ABOUT THE POSE:

This pose activates the feminine lunar energy, which is the balance of the fiery masculine energy of the sun. With too much fire energy, we burn out because we cannot find calm and serenity. We need both energies to find balance.

BODY BENEFITS:

In Half Moon Pose the whole body is coordinated in all areas—the pose strengthens the ankles, thighs, butt, and abdomen while stretching the calves, hamstrings, and groin and opening the hips, torso, chest, and shoulders. Since Half Moon is a mild inversion like Downward-Facing Dog, it causes blood to rush to the brain, providing some of the same benefits of relieving fatigue, stress, and anxiety.

PROPS:

Before you begin, place a block outside a wide-legged stance. When you come into the pose, your hand will drop down to rest on the block. Alternatively you can hold on to the block as you drop the arm down, placing the block on the floor mid-pose. You can also place that hand on the seat of a chair to get a little more height. If you want some more support as you are learning to balance, stand a half a foot away from a wall so you can lean against it if you start to lose your balance.

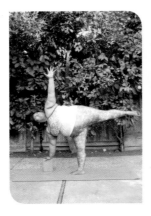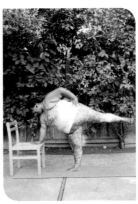

GET IN POSITION:

Stand with feet 2–3 feet apart on your mat facing its long side. Pivot your right foot outward so your toes are pointing to the right. Place your left hand onto your left hip. Bend your right knee, and lean your torso sideways to the right side. Drop your right arm down, placing your hand onto a prop or the floor about 1–2 feet in front of the right foot and just a couple inches to the right.

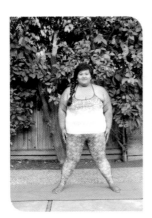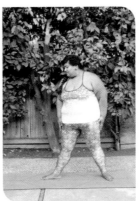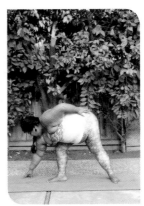

WHEN YOU ARE READY:

Press your fingertips into the prop or the floor and shift the weight of your body over to the right foot. Keep the gaze focused down on the right hand. Lift your left foot 6 inches off the ground, then extend the right leg and establish your balance on your right foot (you can stay here if it feels challenging enough for you. The more you practice, the higher you will be able to lift your leg, until it is parallel to the floor.) Once you find your position for Half Moon Pose, broaden your shoulders, opening up your chest. Push your hips forward. Gaze ahead, focusing on your *drishti* to help with balance.

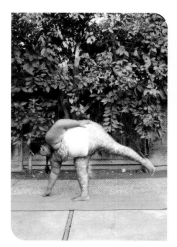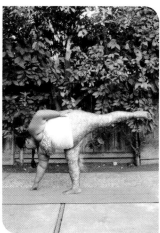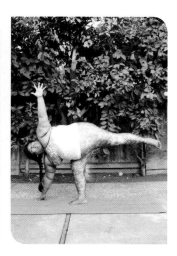

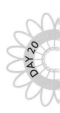

If you feel good here with the hand on the hip, stay here. If you want to challenge yourself more, on the next inhale, reach your left hand up towards the sky, taking your gaze up to your hand. Ground your right hand down so your arms are aligned and perpendicular to the floor. Lengthen from the crown of your head to the sole of your left foot, extending the body. Exit the pose by bringing your left hand back down to your hip, bending the right knee, dropping the left foot down to the floor, and coming back up into an upright position.

HOW LONG:

Hold the pose for 10-30 *ujjayi* breaths, keeping the breath slow, controlled, and steady. Repeat the pose again on the opposite side, holding for another 10-30 *ujjayi* breaths.

REVERSE WARRIOR

(Viparita Virabhadrasana)

ABOUT THE POSE:

Reverse Warrior is a variation of the Warrior 2 posture that is sometimes also called the Dancing Warrior. In a Vinyasa practice, Reverse Warrior comes after Warrior 1 and Warrior 2 as a flow. The pose is fiery and strong, activating the masculine sun energy within us.

BODY BENEFITS:

As in the other warrior series, the lower half of the body is strengthened and stretched. By drawing the arm back in this pose, we stretch the torso, waist, shoulders, and arms. This pose allows more blood to flow throughout the body, which reduces fatigue.

PROPS:

If you struggle with balance, try practicing with a wall by your side. Place your fingertips lightly on the wall to keep you focused in the posture. If you don't have a wall by you, place a chair beside your back leg to hold on to for balance.

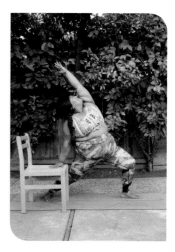

GET IN POSITION:

Begin in a wide-legged stance. Pivot your left foot outward so the toes are pointing to the left, and the heels are aligned with one another. Inhale and raise both arms up and overhead. Exhale, dropping the arms out to the sides, so they are parallel to the floor with palms facing down and bend the left knee so it is over the ankle with the shin perpendicular to the floor. Drop the tailbone down, opening up your hips into Warrior 2.

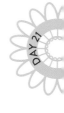

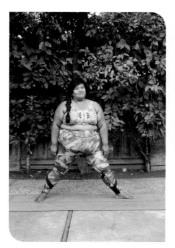

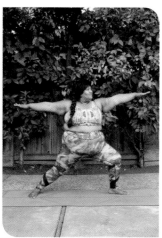

WHEN YOU ARE READY:

Place your right hand on the back of your right thigh or on a chair close to your thigh. Raise your left arm up and back, reaching your fingertips and the crown of your head up to the sky. Lengthen your spine with a slight arch in your back, and sink your hips down.

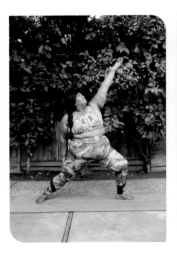 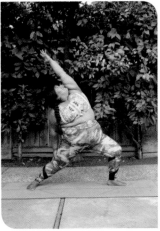

HOW LONG:

Hold for 10–30 *ujjayi* breaths, feeling the fire energy build within the body. Repeat on the opposite side.

EXTENDED SIDE ANGLE POSE

(Utthita Parsvakonasana)

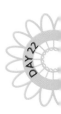

ABOUT THE POSE:

In this pose, all of your muscles are being utilized, building strength within the whole body. This can be a deep hip-opening posture, so take your time working yourself deeper into the pose.

BODY BENEFITS:

This pose strengthens the legs, ankles, groin, chest, lungs, shoulders, spine, and abdomen. It can be used for therapeutic purposes like relieving lower backache, sciatica, menstrual discomfort, and constipation.

PROPS:

When practicing Extended Side Angle, there are a handful of different arm positions to try depending on what feels best to you. One position places the hand down on the ground. If you find reaching the ground difficult, place a block down by the inside of your foot, so when you drop your hand down it will be supported higher up on the block. You can also replace the block with a chair if you can't go deeper into the pose yet. When working on your balance, stand facing away from a wall so you know it's there for support behind you if you lose your balance.

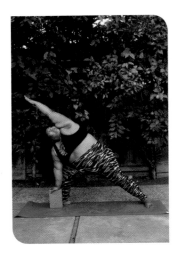

GET IN POSITION:

Begin in a wide-legged stance lengthwise on your mat. Pivot your right foot outward, keeping your heels aligned with each other. Keep your torso facing ahead as you bend your right knee so it is aligned over your right ankle, bringing your right thigh as parallel to the floor as you can.

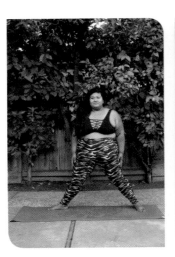
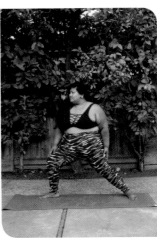
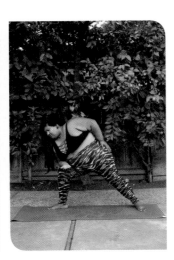

WHEN YOU ARE READY:

Place your right elbow down on top of your thigh with your fingers spread wide and palm facing up like you are holding a platter. Alternatively you can drop the hand down to the floor or prop next to the inner or outer part of the right foot. Inhale and sweep your left arm up and over, palm facing down, to create a straight line with the left leg. Feel the long stretch from the fingertips of your left hand, down your arm and left side of your body, all the way down the left leg and grounded left foot. Open your chest by pushing the torso towards the front, gazing ahead or up at the left hand. Exit the pose by sweeping the left arm back and coming back up to a wide-legged stance.

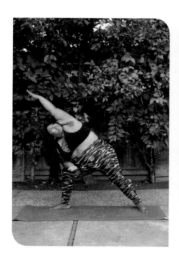
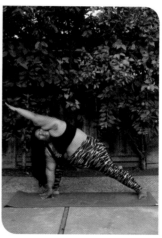
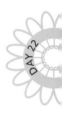

HOW LONG:

Hold for 10–30 *ujjayi* breaths. Repeat on the left side and hold for another 10–30 *ujjayi* breaths.

VARIATION:

Revolved Side Angle Pose—Begin in Extended Side Angle Pose with your elbow resting on your thigh. Drop your extended hand down and place onto the floor or prop inside your bent knee's foot. Once you have established balance, twist your torso and take your gaze back behind you, and sweep the arm that was resting on your thigh up and overhead. Reach out to make a long straight line all the way from the tips of the fingers, down the arm, across the twisted torso, down the hip, and into the back foot grounded to the floor. Hold for 10–30 breaths. Practice this right after the regular Extended Side Angle Pose, before you repeat on the opposite side.

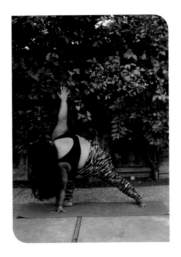

DAY 23

BOW POSE

(Danurasana)

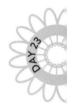

ABOUT THE POSE:

Bow Pose is a deep backbend mimicking an archer's bow. The torso, pelvis, and legs make the arch, and the arms create the string.

BODY BENEFITS:

While strengthening the back muscles, Bow Pose also stretches the whole front of your body—throat, chest, abdomen, hip flexors, groin, quadriceps, and ankles. This pose improves poor posture from hunching over a desk all day and creates flexibility in the spine. By balancing on the pelvic area, you stimulate your digestive and reproductive organs, which can relieve constipation and menstrual cramps.

PROPS:

When first practicing Bow Pose, it might be difficult to grab ahold of both of your ankles. Before getting onto your stomach, loop one strap around both ankles, or two straps around each ankle, and lay the straps down beside your hips as you lie down on your stomach. Grab ahold of the strap(s), walking your hands up the straps as far as you can. Using the straps helps by giving you some extra reach.

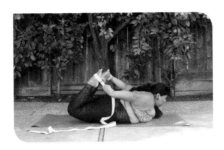

GET IN POSITION:

Begin by lying flat on your stomach with your chin down on the mat and arms down by your sides or out in front. Bend your knees, bringing your heels close to your butt. Grab on to the outer ankles or strap(s) one at a time. Once you have a good grip, bring your knees about hip-width apart, flex your feet, and drop your forehead down to the mat.

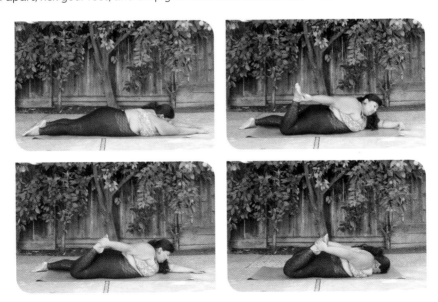

WHEN YOU ARE READY:

Inhale and raise your head, gazing at a point ahead. Lightly lift your chest up off the mat, keeping your thighs flat on the ground. Lift the soles of your feet and the crown of your head up as the pelvis and stomach ground down. If this feels like a good place to stay, stay here. To keep going deeper into the pose, lift your chest higher up off the ground, pull your shoulders back, and elongate your neck by reaching up with the crown of your head. Ground your pelvis onto the mat, lift your knees off the ground, and flex your feet, lifting up the soles.

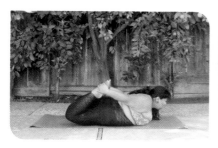 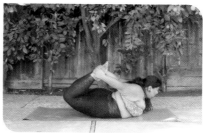

HOW LONG:

Hold for 10–30 *ujjayi* breaths, keeping your breath slow and deep through your belly.

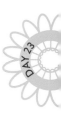

VARIATIONS:

Half Bow—If you want to practice Bow Pose one side at a time before you go for the Full Bow, grab on to your outer right ankle or strap with the right hand and bring your left arm out in front of you. As you would in a regular Bow Pose, inhale and lift up your chest, head, and thighs off the ground. Your right side will be in a Half Bow Pose, and the left arm and leg will be reaching up and out. Hold for 10–30 breaths, coming back down switching legs, and repeating again on the opposite side.

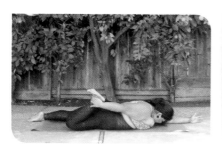 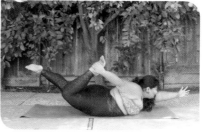

PIGEON POSE

(Eka Pada Rajakapotasana)

ABOUT THE POSE:

The pigeon can represent a number of things like a good sense of direction, homecoming, or puffing out your chest in pride. While you're practicing this pose think of the proud pigeon and feel proud of your body and yourself.

BODY BENEFITS:

Practicing this pose every day can slowly chip away at the years of built-up tension. It stretches the muscles of the thighs, groin, and abdomen, while helping lessen the pain of sciatica, relieve tension in the chest and shoulders, and stimulate the abdominal organs to help with digestion.

PROPS:

When practicing Pigeon it will take a while for your hips to open up enough to allow your pelvis to rest on the floor. Until then, you can place a block, rolled-up blanket, or bolster underneath the upper thigh or hip of your front leg. Adjust the prop to whatever position makes you feel comfortable.

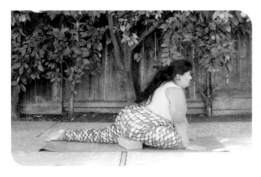
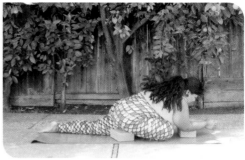

One way to practice Pigeon off the floor is to use a small table, a regular-size table, a bench, or the edge of your bed. If you are using a table, push it against a wall so the opposite side is supported. Stand in front of your prop, lift your left knee placing it onto the edge, then swing the left foot up onto the prop. The left knee, shin, ankle, and foot should be resting at the edge of your prop. Place your hands down next to the knee and foot, push and lift your torso upright, sinking the hips down, while pressing into the floor with your right foot, shifting the right foot back if you want to go a little deeper.

GET IN POSITION:

Begin on all fours, with your wrists underneath your shoulders and your knees underneath your hips. Move your left knee up to your left wrist, and swing your left ankle under your right hip or next to your right wrist. Find out which position works for you.

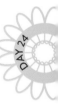

DAY 24

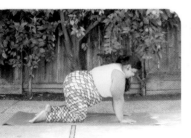
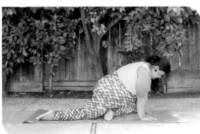
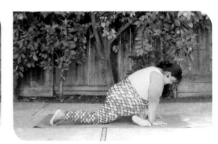

WHEN YOU ARE READY:

Wiggle and slide your right leg straight back, inching it farther back and opening the hips. Sink your hips and pelvis down towards the floor, placing a prop underneath your left hip for support if needed. Place your hands in front of your left shin or by the side of your hips, rooting them into the floor. Push your chest out and elongate your spine, lifting up from your tailbone to the crown of your head.

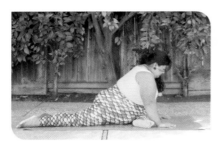
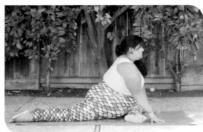

HOW LONG:

Hold for 10 seconds to 1 minute, keeping a steady and controlled *ujjayi* breath. This is a good pose in which to take your time to sit and feel the hips opening up. Exit the pose by scooting the right leg forward, lifting your hips back up, and returning to all fours. Then repeat on the opposite side.

VARIATIONS:

Restorative Pigeon—For a more restorative variation, begin in Pigeon Pose, then walk your hands forward and drape your torso over your front shin. Your arms can be out in front, or elbows and forearms down supporting the torso. You can use a bunch of props to help you relax into this pose such as a bolster or two to create a slope to rest your torso over. Hold for 3–5 minutes.

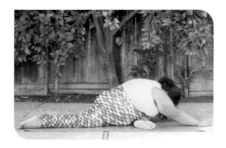

One-Legged King Pigeon—A deeper backbend version of Pigeon Pose is the King Pigeon. This variation is a backbend and hip opener. A strap is recommended when you first practice this pose because it will take time to go deeper into the backbend. The strap helps make the hand-and-foot connection. Loop and tighten a strap around the foot of the leg that will be behind you. Begin in Pigeon Pose, bend the back leg's knee, grab on to the strap, and reach both arms straight back, slightly dropping the head back. You want to gradually walk the hands down the strap to as far as your back will let you towards the back foot, creating a triangular space between the back, leg, and arms. It will take time to eventually grab ahold of the back foot with your hand. Hold for 5–30 *ujjayi* breaths and repeat on the opposite side.

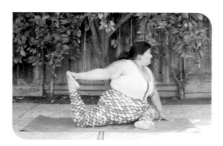

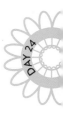

Mermaid Pose—A more advanced variation of One-Legged King Pigeon is Mermaid Pose. Begin in Pigeon Pose with your back knee bent and foot in the air. Hold on to your ankle and pull your foot towards your butt. As you bring the foot closer in, hook the front of the foot with your forearm—eventually you will be able to hook the foot in the inner elbow. Inhale and raise your other arm up overhead. Bend your elbow, dropping your hand behind your head, and grab on to the hand that is hooking your foot. This intensifies the backbend quality of this pose.

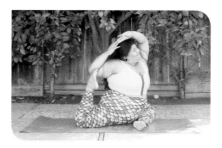

LIZARD AND HALF MONKEY

(Utthan Pristhasana and Ardha Hanumanasana)

ABOUT THE POSE:

The hips and pelvis are the foundational parts of alignment in *asana* practice. Opening the hips helps to release so much stuck tension that can give us problems on a daily basis. Lizard Pose is another great deep hip opener. Half Monkey is the first step in preparing for full Monkey Pose, a.k.a the splits. Monkey Pose is a full-frontal split named after the monkey God Hanuman, who took one huge step reaching from the farthest shore of India to the shore of Sri Lanka. Half Monkey is the beginning of this deep split.

BODY BENEFITS:

Even though Lizard Pose and Pigeon Pose may look similar, Lizard shifts the stretch from the quadriceps to the hamstring. This is a good pose to help with hip flexibility and strengthening the leg muscles.

Beginning in Half Monkey and moving towards the full Monkey Pose will start to open up the hamstrings, quadriceps, groin, and hip flexors while stretching the front and back of your legs.

PROPS:

For Lizard Pose place blocks down between your hands as you begin the pose on all fours or in Downward-Facing Dog position. Your forearms or hands rest on top of the blocks to give a little more height if you are still working on going deeper into the pose. If being down on the floor is difficult for you, use a low table, bench, or the edge of a low bed to practice higher up. Stand 2–3 feet away and place one foot on the edge of your prop and bend your knee. Drop your hands or forearms down to the prop next to the inner ankle. You will still get the deep stretch in the hamstrings without having to be on the floor.

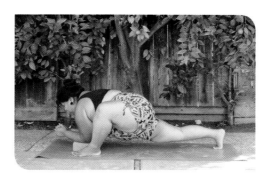

In Half Monkey hold on to those blocks from Lizard and place them next to your sides to bring the floor up to you. To come into Half Monkey from Lizard Pose with either a low table, bench, or low bed, shift your hips back, extending the bent front leg straight with your foot on your prop. Your torso should fold over the front thigh, as your hands support your knee joint.

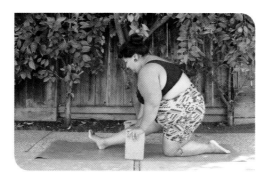

DAY 25

GET IN POSITION:

There are two ways to begin in Lizard Pose depending on your level of flexibility. An easier way of entering the pose is to begin standing at the front of your mat and taking a big step back, 3–4 feet, with the right foot. Bend your left knee and drop your hands down to the inside of your front ankle and lift your back knee off the ground. The intermediate way of entering the pose is by beginning in Downward-Facing Dog (see Day 10). Lift one leg up into a Three-Legged Downward-Facing Dog, then sweep the foot down and forward between your hands. This motion can be done in multiple steps. The sweeping motion is meant to give more leverage when bringing the foot forward.

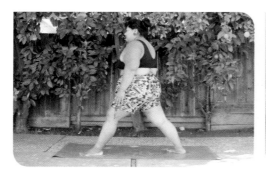
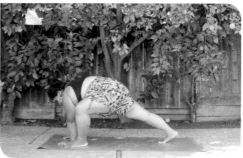

WHEN YOU ARE READY:

Drop down to your forearms on the floor or blocks with your elbows aligned with the heel of your front foot, forearms straight, and palms down with fingers spread wide. Press down with your forearms, lifting up your chest. Keep your back flat and in a straight line from the crown of your head, down your back, through your back leg, and into the ball of your grounded foot.

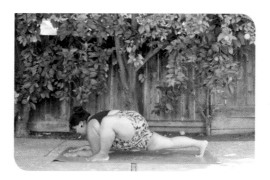

TRANSITIONING TO HALF MONKEY:

From Lizard Pose, drop your back knee down to the floor, come back onto the hands, and shift your hips back as your front leg extends, sitting over your heel with your front foot flexed. Place your hands down by your sides on the floor. This shifts the stretch to the front leg, preparing it for a full Monkey Pose.

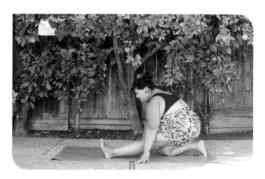

HOW LONG:

Hold Lizard Pose for 10-30 *ujjayi* breaths and then Half Monkey Pose for 10-30 *ujjayi* breaths. Keep your breath slow and steady. Repeat Lizard and Half Monkey again on the opposite sides.

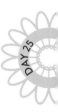

VARIATION:

Monkey Pose (*Hanumanasana*)—Practicing a full Monkey Pose or the splits takes a while to work up to. Don't be in a hurry to jump into the pose. Your muscles need to fully warm up with constant repetition of practice. Before attempting Monkey Pose, practice at least 5 rounds of Lizard and Half Monkey on each side, taking your time to let your muscles warm and stretch. If you feel like your body is ready to start practicing Monkey Pose, grab your props as an added help. Also practicing on a slick surface helps a lot. A slick surface helps by allowing the feet to slide apart more easily. If you are on a sticky mat, your feet won't slide as well.

Begin in a Half Monkey position with your left leg out in front with heel on the floor and your hands on the ground or up on blocks. Slide or wiggle your left heel forward and your right leg backward. Your hips should be aligned next to each other, and not one in front of the other. Place a block underneath your upper left thigh or sit bones to help support your pelvis. Find the limit of how deep you can go. If you are in pain, rise up and lessen the deepness of the stretch. You should be comfortable but challenged as you feel the stretch in your thighs and pelvis.

Your torso should be lengthened from the tailbone up, and angled forward. After some practice, when you become comfortable "sitting" in the pose, bring your torso upright with the crown of your head lifting straight up. Place your hands together at your heart center in prayer hands.

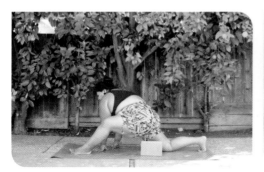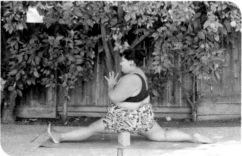

Hold for 10-30 *ujjayi* breaths. To come out of the pose, press your hands into the floor or props, sliding or wiggling your legs back inwards. Come into a Half Monkey. Take a moment to rest the body in a Child's Pose (see Day 9), and repeat on the opposite side.

BRIDGE POSE AND WHEEL POSE

(Setu Bandha Sarvangasana and Chakrasana)

ABOUT THE POSE:

Bridge Pose is a beginning backbend that helps you experiment with the depths of your back-bends. Practicing this pose will help you reach deeper backbends like Wheel Pose, also called Upward Bow.

BODY BENEFITS:

Bridge Pose is considered a mild inversion since the heart is higher than the head, which means it can reduce stress, fatigue, anxiety, headaches, and mild depression. This is a good opener for the chest, heart, and shoulders, while also stretching the back of the neck, spine, hip flexors, and thighs. It also stimulates the thyroid glands to regulate metabolism and digestion.

In addition, Wheel Pose stretches the shoulders, chest, spine, upper back, and thighs while strengthening the wrists, arms, spine, abdomen, and legs. This deep backbend opens up the chest and lungs to help you breathe deeply.

PROPS:

If you would like a little help keeping your hips up off the ground in Bridge Pose or want a more restorative modification, place one or more blocks or a bolster underneath the spot where your lower back and upper butt meet (the sacrum) and rest the weight of your body against the prop.

After practicing Bridge Pose for a while, you can also play around with a yoga wheel. Begin by sitting on the floor with your knees bent and feet on the floor. Place the wheel at the base of your spine and slowly push back with your feet, rolling your spine up and over the wheel while extending your legs. Roll all the way back, placing your head, neck, and shoulders down on the floor. Your shoulders should press into the floor supporting the rest of your body.

Wheel Pose is considered an intermediate to advanced pose, so if you are still new to yoga *asana*, lying over two sturdy chairs is an approachable way of practicing till you feel comfortable entering the pose in the way that I explain later. Place two sturdy chairs facing each other and butted up. You can place a folded blanket over the seam of the chairs for cushioning. Sit at the edge in between the chairs holding on to the backrests. Slowly lower your back over the blanket, letting the chest open up and head hang over the edge on one side and the legs on the other side. Let your arms reach back, resting the tops of the hands on the floor (if possible). Grab on to the backrests to help pull yourself back up into a seated position.

GET IN POSITION:

Begin on your mat, lying down on your back. Bend your knees, keeping them hip-distance apart, and place your feet down on the floor, bringing the heels of your feet close to your butt. Place your arms at your sides, palms facing down. Add your prop here if needed.

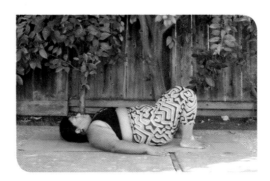

WHEN YOU ARE READY:

Press your hands and feet down into the mat. Lift your pelvis up towards the sky, bringing your butt up off the ground to raise the hips up. You should feel your butt firm, but not squeeze. Press your hands, arms, and shoulders into the mat to support your hips. Alternatively, roll your shoulders back, bringing your shoulder blades closer together, and clasp your hands underneath your back. Your feet should be firmly planted and pressing evenly into the mat. Your body should create a gentle arc from the base of your neck, through the spine, thighs, and to your knees.

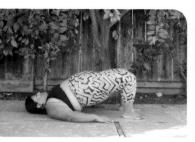 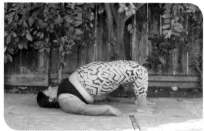 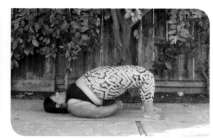

HOW LONG:

Hold for 20 seconds to 1 minute, breathing slowly and steadily through the lower lungs with your *ujjayi* breath. To come out of the pose, release the arms if they are clasped underneath you, using the hands to support the hips as you lower them down to the floor.

TRANSITION TO WHEEL POSE:

This is a more advanced pose but can still be practiced by a beginner. Begin in your original starting position, bringing your heels a little closer to your butt. Raise your arms up and over your head, and place your hands, palms down, on the floor above your shoulders with your fingertips pointing towards your body, and your elbows pointing upward. Lift your pelvis, bringing your butt up off the ground and supporting yourself up on the shoulders like you would in Bridge Pose. If this feels like a good position for now, stay here. If you want to go farther, press your hands down to lift your shoulders and chest up off the ground. Roll from the base of your skull to the crown of your head. In this pose the body is being supported evenly on five points; the feet, hands, and crown. This can be a tough transition, so take your time, and if you need to stay here this will be your Wheel Pose for now. The last motion in Wheel Pose is achieved by extending your arms straight and lifting your head up off the ground. This is accomplished by a combination of pushing up with the arms and using your core to lift your navel up. Once you are up, make sure your shoulders are aligned over your wrists, or as far as you can manage at the moment. Find an even distribution of weight in the hands and feet, remembering to lift up with the core as you lengthen the spine.

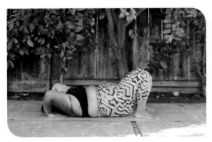 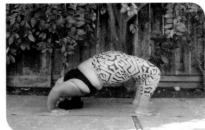 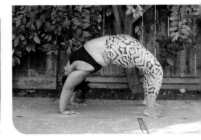

To come out of Wheel, try to refrain from just dropping out of the pose. Steadily drop the crown of your head back down to the floor, and roll your head and shoulders back down to the mat. Bend your knees forward over your toes, drop your back and butt back down, and release your legs and arms back down flat on the mat.

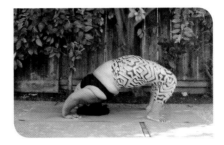

HOW LONG:

This pose requires a lot of strength within the core and arms, which takes constant practice to build up. Hold for 5–60 seconds, remembering to breathe from the lower lungs. The concentration involved in this pose can make you forget to breathe, so keep the breath slow and steady.

FOLLOW-UP:

Since Wheel Pose is a deep backbend, it is good to take time to recover after the pose. Once you've come all the way down to the floor, take a couple moments to lie on your back and catch your breath. Bend your knees, bringing your feet closer to your butt, then drop both knees over to the right side, creating a slight twist. Gaze back over your left shoulder. Repeat on your other side. Bring your knees back to center and hug them to your chest. Rock from side to side to massage your back against the floor. Then come up to finish in a Child's Pose (see Day 9).

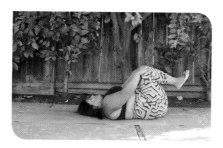

VARIATION:

Forearm Wheel—If being on the wrists in Wheel Pose is too challenging at the moment, begin in the second position for Wheel Pose, supported on the five points. Instead of straightening your arms, drop each arm down to the forearm with your elbows beside your head. The palms can be flat on the floor or clasped together creating a tripod around your head. From here, lift up your navel using your core strength. Extend your legs and align your shoulders over your elbows or as close as you can at the moment. Hold for 10–30 *ujjayi* breaths.

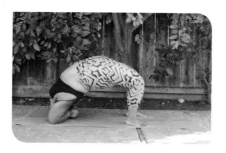

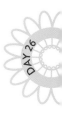

DAY 26

HALF LORD OF THE FISHES POSE

(Ardha Matsyendrasana)

ABOUT THE POSE:

This pose is named after one of the first known yogis, Matsyendra. In old scriptures he was a fish who desired to become human, a wish granted to him by the deity Shiva. This pose represents his evolution from fish to human. While practicing this pose, think about the ways you may want to grow and evolve in your own life, and appreciate the ways in which you already have.

BODY BENEFITS:

Twisting is a good way to transition from backbends to forward bends. It is also good for digestion and stimulating the kidneys and liver. The Lord of the Fishes stretches the shoulders, hips, and spine to help relieve fatigue, backache, and problems from sciatica.

PROPS:

This is a seated posture; if it is difficult to sit flat on the floor because your sit bones roll backward, place a folded blanket underneath your sit bones to prop you up. This will help you to keep an upright position in the pose.

If you would like to practice this sitting on a chair, sit at the edge so as not to use the backrest and place a small step stool or a couple stacked blocks a couple inches away from the chair. Step one foot onto the blocks or step stool so the foot is close to the opposite knee, or rest one foot on top of the opposite thigh.

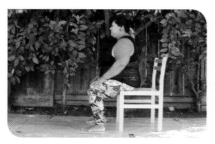 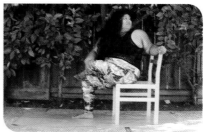

GET IN POSITION:

Begin seated on the floor with your legs out in front of you, and arms down by your sides. There are a few leg positions you can try while practicing this pose. If you are not very flexible yet, bend your left knee, placing your foot next to the inside of your right knee, or try crossing your foot over to the outside of your right knee. See which one feels best for you.

The more advanced version is to bend both knees with the soles of your feet on the floor. Drop your right knee down to the floor, tucking your right leg under your left leg. Bring your right foot under your left buttock and step your left foot to rest the ankle over your right knee with the sole on the floor.

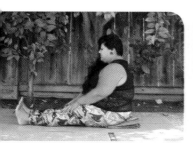 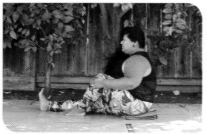 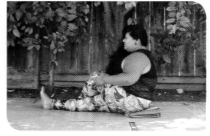

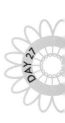

WHEN YOU ARE READY:

Place the left hand down onto the floor behind the left hip. Inhale and raise your right arm. Exhale and twist your upper body to the left side. Drop your right arm down on the outside of your left knee. Your arm can be straight, fingers pointing down towards the floor, hand hooked around your knee, or bent at the elbow and palm facing towards the left. Use your arm as leverage against your knee to twist all the way to the left side. The twist should start from your right hip, spread across your torso, and up your left shoulder, ending with the gaze over the left shoulder.

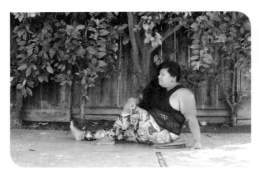 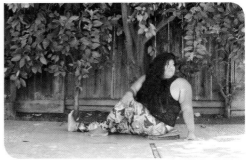

HOW LONG:

Hold for 30 seconds to 1 minute, inhaling and exhaling as you go deeper into the twist just a little more with each breath. Don't push yourself too far into the pose if you are not ready for it. Take your time easing into the twist. Exit the pose and repeat on the opposite side.

FLOW DAYS 15-27 POSES

HOW TO TRANSITION:

Remember this is not a race! Take your time in each position to feel the benefits of each pose. This second set of flow moves the body up and down from pose to pose. The transitions don't have to look pretty, but they can still be practiced fluidly as you transition from one pose to the next.

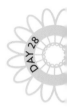

- ✦ Extended Triangle Pose > Goddess Pose
- ✦ Goddess Pose > Garland Pose
- ✦ Garland Pose > Tree Pose
- ✦ Tree Pose > King Dancer Pose
- ✦ King Dancer Pose > Half Moon Pose
- ✦ Half Moon Pose > Reverse Warrior
- ✦ Reverse Warrior > Extended Side Angle Pose

- ✦ Extended Side Angle Pose > (Plank Pose > Four-Limbed Staff Pose) > Bow Pose
- ✦ Bow Pose > Pigeon Pose
- ✦ Pigeon Pose > Lizard Pose
- ✦ Lizard Pose > Half Monkey Pose
- ✦ Half Monkey Pose > Bridge Pose
- ✦ Bridge Pose > Wheel Pose
- ✦ Wheel Pose > (Child's Pose) > Half Lord of the Fishes Pose

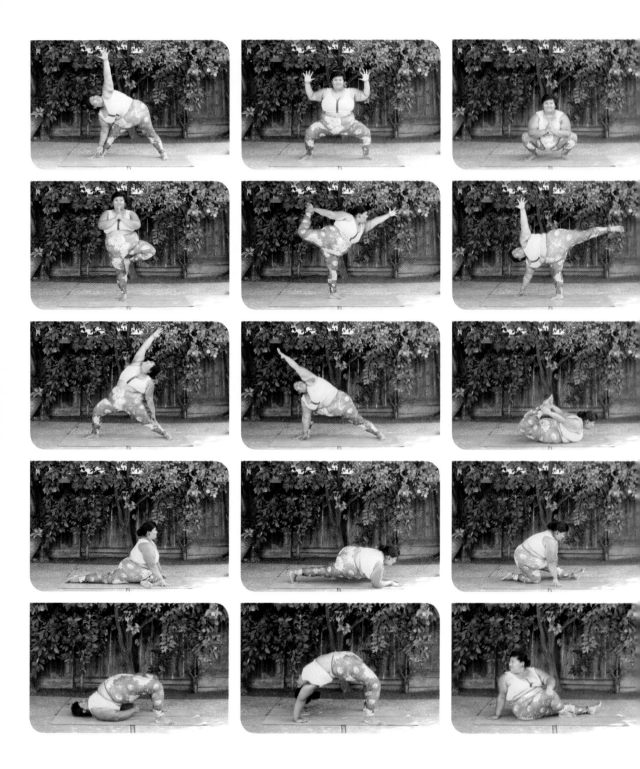

PROPS:

Whenever you are practicing a flow, it is good to have all your props ready for you next to your mat. Even if you don't end up using them, they are there to help you out if you need them. If you know you need a wall, practice next to the wall. Have your chair out and ready, blocks set up on each side of you, one or two straps, blanket or bolsters at the ready.

MAKE ADJUSTMENTS:

If something doesn't feel right, take the time to physically move things around. Sometimes my belly gets in the way when I want to go deeper into a pose, so I lift it up and move it to open up more space. If transitioning from a pose in one big step is difficult, break that big step into smaller steps. Be kind to yourself and your body; we are not all able to adapt to new things quickly. Our bodies have to take time to learn with repeated motions. You are also allowed to stop and drop into a Child's Pose (see Day 9) whenever the buildup of energy is a bit overwhelming. Take a moment to catch your breath and then keep going.

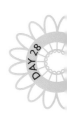

DAY 28

SUPINE SPINAL TWIST

(Supta Matsyendrasana)

ABOUT THE POSE:

Supine Spinal Twist is sometimes referred to as the lying-down version of the Lord of the Fishes Pose. This twist is a great way to wring out the frustrations of a long day and help restore balance. It also stimulates the abdominal muscles to aid in digestion and the release of toxins.

BODY BENEFITS:

This pose lengthens and relaxes the spine as it stretches the back muscles and glutes. As you twist, your abdominal muscles, back, and hips all get a massage.

PROPS:

Using a strap in this position is the best because it lets you just enjoy the pose without worrying about whether you can reach your hand to your foot. A strap lets you get the full twist with the extended leg. It can be looped in two ways: one way is to hold each end of the strap and place your foot in the middle, looping the strap around the ball of your foot. The second way is to make a loop from the buckle end of your strap, tightening it around the ball of your foot.

GET IN POSITION:

Begin lying on your back with your arms down by your sides. If you are not using a strap, bend both of the knees into the chest. With the strap, bend your right knee, hugging it into your chest, and loop the strap around the ball of the foot. With the strap, extend your right leg up so that it is perpendicular to the floor, holding the strap in your left hand.

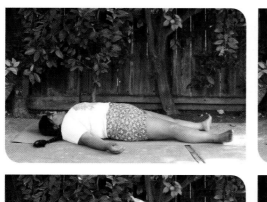
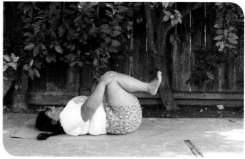
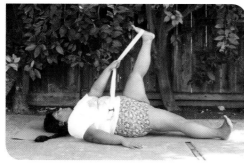
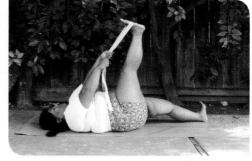

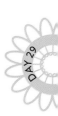

WHEN YOU ARE READY:

Without the strap, drop both knees over to the left side, and turn the torso and chest over to-wards the right side, dropping the arms down and out into a "T," looking at the right hand. Using the strap, cross your right leg over to the left side of your body, twisting your torso, and drop or hover your leg down over to the left side. Drop your right shoulder and arm down with your fin-gertips pointing to the right. Turn your head and gaze over to the right side. Feel the twist all the way from your right arm, across your chest and torso, and down your right hip, leg, and foot.

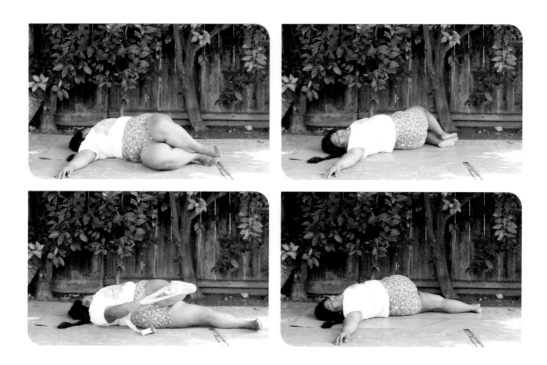

HOW LONG:

Hold for 30 seconds to a couple minutes. This is a great pose to just sink into and relax in. Enjoy every bit of it. Exit the pose by bringing your knees or leg back up and switching to practice on the opposite side.

DAY 30

BOUND ANGLE POSE

(Baddha Konasana)

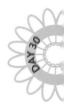

ABOUT THE POSE:

Bound Angle Pose is a hip opener that can be practiced throughout the day to help relieve tension and stiffness in the hips from poor posture. The restorative variation of bound angle gives a gentle backbend of this pose to open up your heart, so use it to practice some self-love.

BODY BENEFITS:

This pose can improve the circulation of blood flow throughout the whole body, especially the pelvis, which helps with symptoms of menstrual pain and menopause. The hips, groin, inner thighs, and knees are all stretched, which can help with sciatic pain.

PROPS:

In any seated position like Bound Angle Pose, you can place a folded or rolled-up blanket underneath the sit bones for added comfort, keeping the spine upright so the lower spine doesn't round.

GET IN POSITION:

Begin sitting on the floor with your legs extended out in front of you, and your hands down by your sides.

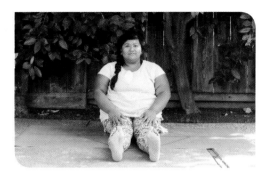

WHEN YOU ARE READY:

Bend your knees, bringing the heels of your feet in towards your pelvis. Drop your knees down on both sides, bringing the soles of your feet together. Only bend your knees and bring the feet in towards the pelvis as far as feels comfortable, while still keeping your knees close to the floor. Press your feet together and hold on to the tops of your feet. Sit upright, lengthening your spine. Lift up with the crown of your head and feel your sit bones root down to the floor.

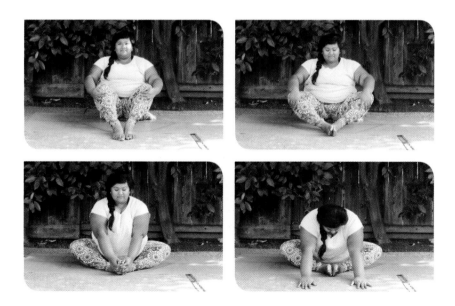

HOW LONG:

Hold the pose for 30 seconds to a couple minutes. Your breath should be calm and steady as you gaze ahead softly.

VARIATION:

Reclined Bound Angle Pose—A nice way to finish this practice is with a Reclined Bound Angle Pose using a bolster, rolled-up blanket, or extra mat. If you don't have these props you can lie with your back resting on the floor. Place your prop end behind your back at the base of your tailbone. Lie back, draping your spine over your prop. This will give a gentle supported back-bend. Let your shoulders and arms drop to each side with your palms up. Feel your heart open up. Hold for 1–3 minutes, letting yourself relax into the pose.

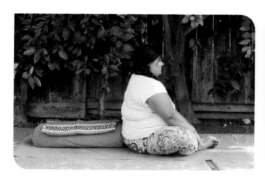
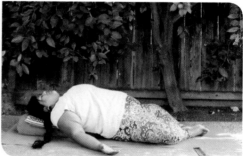
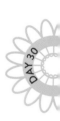

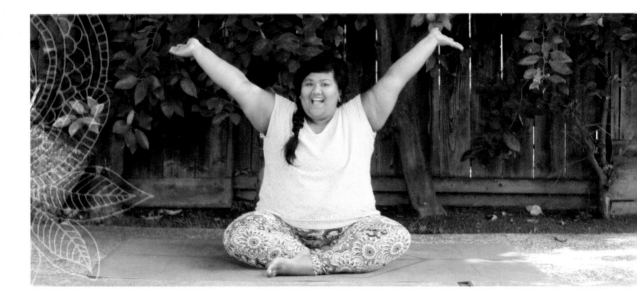

YOU MADE IT!

Congratulations! I'm glad that you made it through the whole challenge. Whether it was easy or difficult, yoga is always about the journey. Reflect on how you felt before you started, and how you feel now. Do you notice a big difference in the way your body feels, or how your mood might have changed? Are you feeling less stressed, more flexible, or pretty much the same? If you took the challenge again, what might you do differently?

I hope this experience has been a positive one, especially for the way you look at life. Remember, this challenge was just the beginning, and if you enjoyed the challenge, keep going!

MORE YOGA FLOW SEQUENCES

Your next yoga goal is to link all of the 30-day challenge poses together. The most obvious sequence is to do these in order, in one yoga session. Take your time transitioning from pose to pose. There doesn't need to be a rush to see how fast you can get through them. Be aware in each position and fully feel the benefits of each posture. Start your practice slowly and at your own speed, then gradually pick up the pace to bring more movement and energy into your practice.

The following suggestions are other sequences you might enjoy:

1 Sun Salutation

+ Mountain Pose (page 82)
+ Standing Backbend (page 86)
+ Forward Fold (page 89)
+ Low Lunge (page 94)
+ Downward-Facing Dog (page 110)
+ Plank Pose or Four-Limbed Staff Pose (page 98)

+ Cobra Pose (page 102)
+ Downward-Facing Dog (page 110)
+ Low Lunge (page 94)
+ Forward Fold (page 89)
+ Standing Backbend (page 86)
+ Mountain Pose (page 82)

2 Energizing the Back

+ Side Stretch and Waist Rotation (page 74)
+ Cat Pose and Cow Pose (page 79)
+ Tiger Pose (page 81)
+ Palm Tree Pose (page 82)

+ Standing Backbend (page 86)
+ Forward Fold (page 89)
+ Chair Pose (page 122)
+ Crescent Lunge (page 97)

3 Hip Opening

+ Bound Angle Pose (page 181)
+ Low Lunge (page 94) and High Lunge (page 97)
+ Lizard Pose (page 162)

+ Pigeon Pose (page 158)
+ Wide-Legged Forward Fold (page 118)
+ Half Lord of the Fishes Pose (page 172)

4 Back Bending

+ Cat Pose and Cow Pose (page 79)
+ Puppy Pose (page 113)
+ Cobra Pose (page 102)

+ Bow Pose (page 155)
+ Bridge Pose (page 167)
+ Wheel Pose (pages 169–170)

⑤ Stress Relieving

+ Reclined Bound Angle Pose (page 183)
+ Child's Pose (page 106)
+ Forward Fold (page 89)
+ Extended Triangle Pose (page 128)
+ Dolphin Pose (page 113)
+ Bridge Pose (page 167)
+ Downward-Facing Dog (page 110)

⑥ Strengthening

+ Leg lifts (pages 76–77)
+ Downward-Facing Dog (page 110)
+ Chair Pose (page 122)
+ Extended Side Angle Pose (page 151)
+ Forearm Plank (page 101)

⑦ Anxiety Reducing

+ Reclined Bound Angle Pose (page 183)
+ Child's Pose (page 106)
+ Forward Fold (page 89)
+ Legs up the wall (page 77)
+ Supported Bridge Pose (page 168)
+ Supine Spinal Twist (page 178)
+ Lying on the floor on your back
+ Tree Pose (page 139)

⑧ Self-Love

+ Standing Backbend (page 86)
+ Wide-Legged Forward Fold (page 118)
+ Goddess Pose (page 132)
+ Half Moon Pose (page 145)
+ Downward-Facing Dog (page 110)
+ Pigeon Pose (page 158)
+ Supine Spinal Twist (page 178)
+ Lying down hugging the knees to chest (page 171)

AERIAL YOGA

Another way to shake up your yoga routine is to leave your mat entirely. In Aerial Yoga, you move through a series of postures while being held up with a hammock that is attached to a sturdy beam or pipe on the ceiling or even a door frame. The hammock supports the body partially or fully, lifting you off the ground. Aerial yoga can be practiced either at home or in a specialized yoga studio.

When I first heard of aerial yoga, it sounded like fun, and I definitely wanted to try out a class. However, I was a little hesitant because as with rock climbing, I thought there would be an issue of whether or not the fabric of the hammock could support my weight. I made sure to check at my local studio that their hammocks could support me without ripping or tearing. To my great relief, I discovered that the bar that connects the hammock to the ceiling can support up to 1,000 pounds, and the fabric itself can support up to 300 pounds. These values may vary from studio to studio and quality of the fabric, but knowing the facts before going helped me feel a lot more confident about trying it out. I am under 300 pounds, so I felt comfortable knowing that I would be completely supported the moment my feet left the ground.

The class was a completely new experience. The hammocks, known as silks, are really just another type of prop, but they require a lot of strength to use them. You still have to rely more on your body than on them. The silks are there to move you, hold you up, and challenge you even more. There were traditional poses and supported poses, and eventually we did hang upside down in the hammocks, which was a lot of fun.

I had to make accommodations for my bigger belly at times. When we were ready to do the hanging poses, the teacher showed me how to wrap the silks under my belly in a way that it would be comfortable. When you are hanging, you are trying to work with gravity and you will feel all of your weight being pressed down onto you. The key is to figure out how you can allow your body to hang upside down in the right spots so it feels comfortable.

I have done inversions before, but I've never done this kind of naturally upside-down yoga, which was really fun and interesting. In one of the poses, you wrap the silk around your back, then fall back slightly and wrap your legs around the sling.

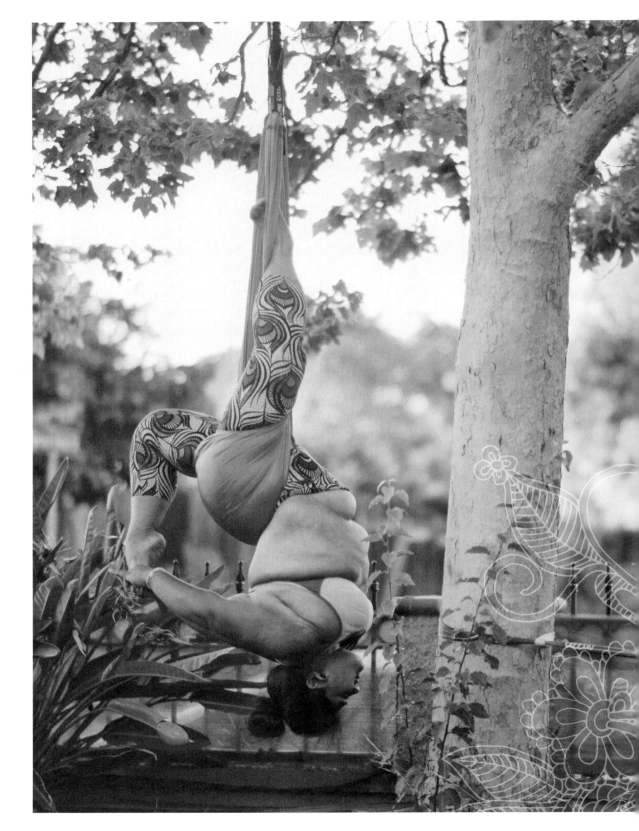

You'd be completely upside down, with your legs supported, hooked into the sling, and then supported by your lower back.

Truth be told, some parts were a little bit painful; it wasn't easy to get over the sensation of the sling pushing in places that I wasn't used to. The hammock is something that I needed to adjust to, both physically and mentally. Even though they are able to hold a bigger-bodied person, you can still feel the fabric moving around you. Sometimes it felt awesome, and sometimes it just plain hurt. It took a bit of trial and error until I could find the right spot and make the necessary modifications for my body in order to make the practice comfortable. For example, when I folded forward over the silks, they landed on the front of my pelvis. This was uncomfortable because of the additional pressure on that area. I was offered the option of adding a blanket into the silks to give them a little more cushion, but

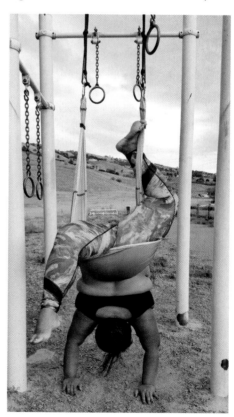

it didn't help me out that much. However, when the class was about halfway through I felt my pelvis go a bit numb and it didn't hurt anymore. By the end it was satisfying floating around the room upside down!

I recommend that first-time practitioners should try it at a specialized yoga studio. My teacher was helpful and understanding. She made me feel comfortable and not singled out in class and assisted me when I was having trouble in some of the postures. I felt much more secure knowing that there was someone spotting me.

If you try it at a studio and feel comfortable, you can move your aerial practice to your home and work out by yourself. The silks and the door supports can be purchased online. I have an Aerial Yoga Trapeze from Yoga Body Naturals (www .yogabody.com). The support needs to be drilled into a door frame, and then hooks on top of the frame itself so it's able to hold your body weight. The sling then hangs from the frame, which is similar to a pull-up bar.

I didn't have a door-frame mount, so I tried it out at a park that had a fitness pull-up bar as part of an exercise circuit. That was strong and sturdy and could definitely hold my weight. I was a bit nervous to be upside down in a public park, but I found an isolated spot where I felt comfortable exposing my tummy. In the end, it was a liberating experience.

Yoga Body Naturals also has a travel metal yoga trapeze stand as well. It can be set up in a room, backyard, or out at a park. I definitely want to try one of those out!

ACRO YOGA

There are tons of images these days of people doing yoga—on the Internet and in popular magazines—that look like a tryout for Cirque Du Soleil. Handstands, back-bends, and pretzeling, oh my! Even for an experienced yogi like me, these pictures can be a little intimidating.

Yet I'm open to trying anything once, especially when it comes to yoga. I've found that Acro Yoga is a fun and playful way to interact with others. Most of the time yoga involves a deeper, inward connection to yourself, but Acro Yoga creates a connection between you and a partner through movement. *Acro* means "high," or "elevated," in Greek. As you know, yoga translates to the notion of union, or joining. By combining acrobatics, yoga, and healing arts, Acro Yoga connects two people—or more—into a single yoga practice. In this sense, Acro Yoga removes the solitary quality of yoga, gets you out of your own head, and deepens relationships. It invites practitioners to tap into new and infinite possibilities of communication, trust, and union and helps to dissolve fears.

In Acro Yoga, one person acts as the base and the other is the flyer. The base lies down on their back, suspending the flyer into the air with the base's feet and hands balancing the flyer's hips, shoulders, butt, or hands. Acro requires a lot of trust and strength from both people. It looks so beautiful, fluid, light, and fun to fly around in the air.

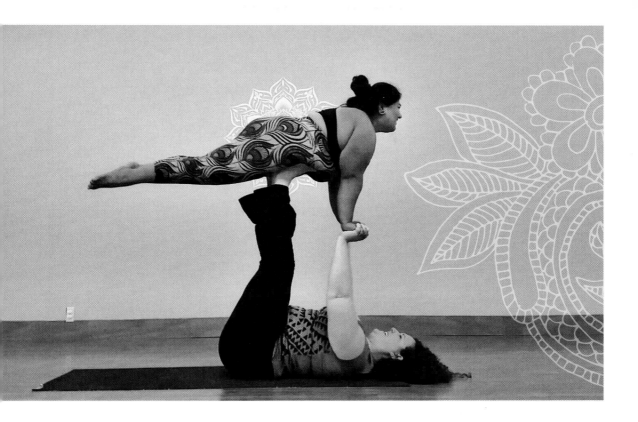

As a bigger-bodied person, being even a small distance off the ground with the chance of falling can be a little nerve racking. I've fallen many times just *standing still*, so putting myself in a position up off the ground seemed pretty unsafe! After all, gravity has the upper hand. I was also afraid that I could hurt somebody, because if they were to lift me up but I wasn't able to hold myself, or they couldn't support me, I could fall and crush them.

Still, I wanted to try it so badly! I craved the sensation of flying, so I gave it a try. I partnered with my friend Naomi, a plus-size yoga teacher from Oakland, California. Naomi is tall and strong, like an Amazon. I felt a little more comfortable because we both have balancing qualities, and she had tried it before with other bigger-bodied people. She definitely has a lot of power. Naomi took the position of base, lying on the floor with her feet in the air. Next, she put her feet on my hips, and we held hands. Then, I shifted my weight over her while she extended her legs out to push me up higher as I extended my arms.

It took a few tries to get it right, but we finally did it. After falling over a whole lot of times, we finally found our balance, and I flew! The feeling was amazing: I was hovering over the ground. I could feel the physical weight of my body pressing down, but I felt free and light. I could only hold the pose for a single minute, but it was an exhilarating minute. Some people can stay up there for 10 or 15 minutes, but I'm happy with my 1 minute.

After my first try, I really had an urge to keep going. The only problem was that Naomi lived an hour away and was really busy with her own schedule. I knew I had another option for a partner, my best friend, Ruel. He and I were already practicing partner yoga together. Being a playful guy, he always liked to prove how strong he was by lifting me up, and I would always be so scared of hurting him that I would ground my feet to the floor so he wouldn't be able to. And, I never felt comfortable just letting him lift me, especially since he is a lot smaller than I am, and there were a lot of trust issues that I had about surrendering myself to someone else.

"For once you have tasted flight you will walk the Earth with your eyes turned skywards, for there you have been and there you will long to return."

—LEONARDO DA VINCI

But after flying my first time, I felt that I was ready to see how it would be with Ruel. Even though he is smaller than I am, he is a strong guy. Practicing Acro Yoga with him still had its challenges. For instance, his feet were a lot smaller than Naomi's, which meant he would be providing me with less surface area to rest on. Normally the base's feet are placed right on the flyer's hip bones so you're balancing evenly, but I am top heavy, so starting low on the hips didn't feel right. We tried many different ways to get me up because it was all just finding what worked for both of us, and eventually it worked. But every time we practice it always feels like the first time, because we are constantly readjusting to one another to find the right groove. We did make it work together, and I was

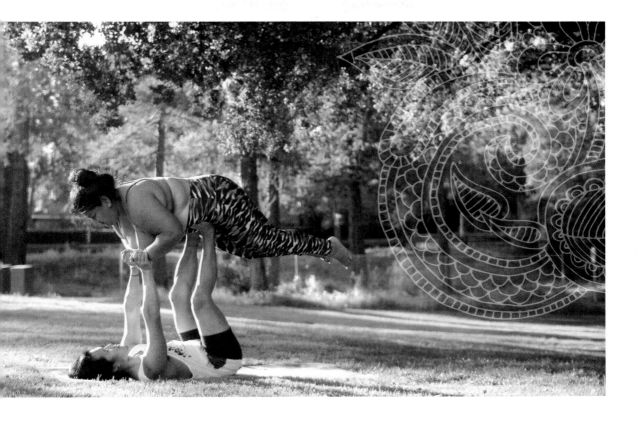

glad that I could get over the fear of overthinking, and just trust in the moment. The most I've done while flying is a one-handed Bird Pose. Bird Pose is the basic Acro Yoga pose where the flyer is being supported only by the base's feet. I'm very happy with what I was able to accomplish in Acro Yoga, and I hope to be able to do a Full Bird Pose one day.

If you want to give Acro a try, first find somebody you trust who's willing to do it with you. Keep in mind that Acro is not really for beginners: you have to have enough experience practicing yoga to have developed some strength and flexibility. It's a more advanced practice, but it is definitely doable for any size or shape. And for your first attempt, I highly recommend doing it in a studio with an instructor who can spot you. An instructor can help guide you, showing you where you need to shift your weight and your balance.

Feeling free and confident in my physical abilities, I can see how far I've come. Being able to trust physically and mentally in someone else has been a huge accomplishment for me, as well.

4

YOU CAN'T CHANGE THE PAST; YOU CAN CHANGE THE FUTURE

YOU CAN'T CHANGE THE PAST; YOU CAN CHANGE THE FUTURE

I don't understand how people can judge me, or anybody else, for stuff that has happened in the past. Having a big body opens you up to criticism, even from people who don't know you well. I've had complete strangers ask me, "Why didn't you eat less when you were younger?" The truth is, there are some parts of our lives that we had little control over, including how our parents treated us in our upbringing, or their beliefs about food and culture. Yet those decisions, good or bad, are part of who we are today.

Every aspect of the woman I am now is a direct result of my past: the influence of my parents, my DNA, the people I've interacted with, what I ate, my environment, my experience, my inner thoughts, others' opinions, family, friends, activities, decisions I've made, events I've gone to, education, and everything in between. At the same time, what has happened in my past is gone and done with, and I'm at peace with it. In fact, I'm grateful for it, and the lessons I learned will continue to carry me into my future. Today, I don't have guilt, and I'm just living my life as I am.

> "The past, like the future, is indefinite and exists only as a spectrum of possibilities."
>
> —STEPHEN HAWKING

While I can't change the past, I'm hopeful about the future. Just because you are the way you are right now doesn't mean that you can't be mentally or physically different tomorrow. There's so much that changes, even within the span of a year, that can influence who you are and who you can be. As long as you have the mindset that you can change—mentally, physically, or emotionally—then you can.

Yoga has helped me jump over mental hurdles that I have placed in front of my own self. It's helped me change for the better and understand that I don't have to give a crap about what other people think about me. That doesn't mean I no longer have insecurities; I just try not to dwell on them. Instead, I can revel in the power of my mind and body.

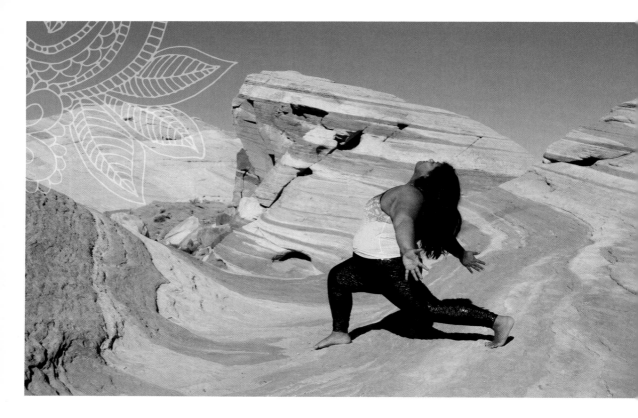

When we come onto our mats to practice, we leave what happened in the past behind us and refrain from thoughts of what will happen in the future. The point of the practice is to bring yourself into the present. Use your time on the mat to forget everything that you had to deal with before coming into a class. Just take your time to be in the present, in the moment, and bask in some positivity for just a little while.

Yoga also has a timeless quality that speaks to change. You're constantly improving every time you practice. The more you can embrace yoga philosophy, the more you can move away from past hurts. Yoga teaches that there is no such thing as perfection: we're simply striving to be better in the future.

DON'T PUT YOUR LIFE ON HOLD

Let's face it—on TV, in ads, and on the Internet, it's difficult to find imagery of bigger-bodied people doing anything that doesn't revolve around weight loss. Before my journey to yoga, I was feeling frustrated about this lack of positive representation until I came across a website of big women doing fun activities like exploring fashion, climbing, surfing, yoga, and other things I had always wanted to do. This was just amazing! These activities had always interested me, but I'd told myself to wait until some elusive date when I was slimmer. But here were these awesome women doing things that I had always wanted to do—they weren't waiting, they were doing!

For me, finding that website was a turning point. I had a new perspective. I finally asked my friends to take me rock climbing! Before I was always so discouraged every time they asked me to join in with them to climb because I didn't think that I could physically do it, but it felt good to be excited about finally starting something new! Once I tried rock climbing, I realized that the obstacles holding me back weren't anything other than my own doubt. I had created the hurdle—but I also had the power to jump over it myself.

> "When we love, we always strive to become better than we are. When we strive to become better than we are, everything around us becomes better too."
>
> —PAULO COELHO, *THE ALCHEMIST*

Even though I could be hard on myself mentally for not being outgoing or confident all the time, I'm still lucky to have not beaten myself up so much about my physical look and for being open to trying new physical activities. I've always lived by my own mantra: *"I can't be anyone or anything else than who and what I am."*

I want to practice yoga, travel to new places, dance my butt off, meet new people, rock climb, camp in the wild, bike for the sheer joy of feeling free, play video games just because it's what I like, and express myself. I've learned to be happy in

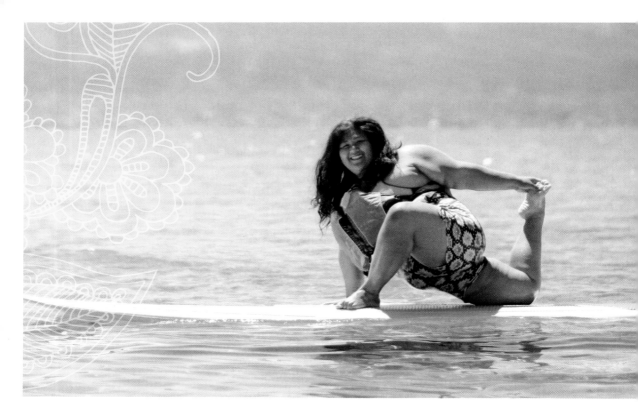

the body that I'm living in *right now*—not next year when I could be thinner. I am mindfully aware of enjoying the present moment.

Try it in your world! Stop focusing on the things you aren't, and commit yourself instead to the things you are and can be. And remember, you won't be able to do everything immediately with ease. We all need to jump or trip over those mental hurdles that we've put upon ourselves. You don't become an expert without struggle and practice—that includes taking on a "go for it" attitude. Give yourself time to embrace the way of life, practice it every day, and I promise you'll see your world widen and you'll have greater joy and contentment.

CONCLUSION

This book describes how I have come to better understand myself through yoga, and I hope you will come to have your own yoga journey as well. Within your own practice, I hope you find a sense of release and an opportunity to enhance your life. There is so much crap that we deal with in this world, we need to find real tools that help us to process out emotion, stay calm, and change the negativity to positivity. These are some of the very important things that yoga provides for me, and I hope it will do the same for you.

Remember, yoga is a practice, and therefore, you must continue to do it in order to get better. There is no "mastering" or an end destination in yoga. Sorry to burst your bubble, but it's really true.

> "Yoga is the journey of the self, through the self, to the self."
>
> —BHAGAVAD GITA

Some people would like to believe that the ultimate goal in yoga is to do a handstand. Yes, that is definitely a cool posture, and will get you some extra "likes" on your social media page, but that's not what yoga is really about. There is no end goal, no destination—just the journey.

Happy travels.

ACKNOWLEDGMENTS

T hank you to my agent Lydia Shamah, ghost writer Pam Liflander, and editor Laura Mazer and her team of amazing people at Seal Press for helping me bring this book to life. If it weren't for you all, this book would still be stuck in my jumbled mind.

To all my friends and family who have cheered me on despite my awkward introverted-ness of receiving praise, I love you all and can't thank you more! This includes both my mom and dad's families (you know I can't name you all because it's a giant-ass Filipino and Mexican family) and my friends who have become my family. Those of you closest to me: Arika, Mikki, Audrey, and Ruel, lots of love.

Thanks to Robin and Peter for letting me use their cabin in North Lake Tahoe to work on big chunks of this book at the beginning of my writing journey. You guys are awesome!

It may sound weird, but thanks to my ex-boyfriend Ryan. We may not have been together long, but I thank you for still being proud, caring, and encouraging of me.

Thanks to my SJSU ceramic and art family for putting up with me for eight years, always asking when I was going to graduate! Art will always be my love, and you guys all made it even better! Much love to Ivan, Allison, Chauncey, Stan, Monica, Ryan, Shannon, Kurt, Ted, Joe, Shelby, Tim, Cassandra, Joey, Yukari, Malia, Wes, Dave, Brittney, Sarah W., and so many other undergrads, BFAs, and MFAs I have met through these years.

Thanks to all the friends, students, and teachers who represent the fact that yoga is for all bodies, in all communities, online and in person.

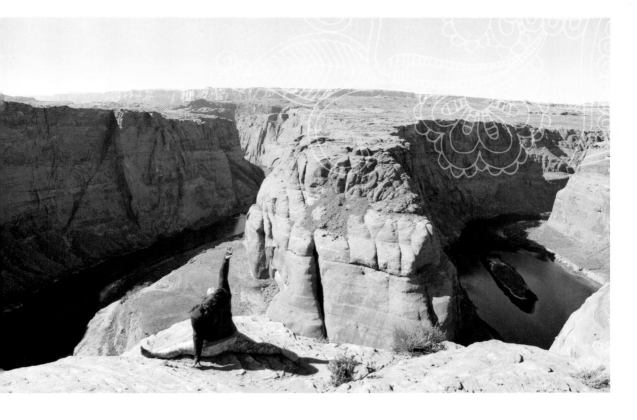

Much love to the owner of Be the Change Yoga and Wellness in downtown San Jose, Taraneh, for being such an amazing friend and for offering an amazing space for the yoga community.

A big thanks to Chrystal Bougon of Curvy Girl Lingerie for offering an amazingly comfortable space for bigger women to feel safe as they embrace their sexual side and offering me a space to connect and teach yoga.

I want to give my love and support to all the inspirational people and communities: body-positive activists, fat femmes, body-positive yoga pioneers, feminists, LGBTQ+, #BlackLivesMatter, indigenous tribes, Latinx and Asian communities, plus-size models, artists, and teachers of all different fields. You all provide us communities in which we can feel comfortable and safe to express ourselves.

And to every fucking amazing beautiful person out there who said they couldn't do something because they were fat—you are worthy of yourself!

ABOUT THE AUTHOR

Valerie Sagun, a.k.a. Big Gal Yoga, is a yoga practitioner, installation artist, ceramicist, radical self-love enthusiast, and body-positive encourager based in San Jose, California. She started college at San Jose State University in 2005 and graduated in 2015 with a Bachelor of Fine Arts in Spatial Arts. There she focused on the hands-on media of ceramics, glass, metals, woodwork, and installation art. During her time at SJSU she took her first yoga class in 2010, where she practiced Hatha Yoga with yogi Lawrence Caughlan. He gave her a positive outlook, teaching her that as long as one has the determination, motivation, and patience, anyone can practice yoga. In January 2016 Valerie attended a Hatha Yoga immersion yoga teacher training at the Seven Centers Yoga Arts Center in Sedona, Arizona. She is now a certified Hatha Yoga teacher, with a private practice where she teaches individuals and groups. Follow Valerie at www.biggalyoga.com or on Instagram @biggalyoga.